Get Your Rear in Gear

GET YOUR
REAR
IN
GEAR

Firming, Toning, and Shaping Your Butt

HARRY HANSON
with Robin K. Levinson

Photos by Jack Linholm

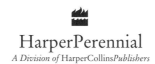

HarperPerennial

A Division of HarperCollins*Publishers*

I dedicate this book to my lovely wife,
Susan Hanson,
the reason I am where I am.
Thank you for your undying support,
love, commitment, and understanding.

HarperCollins books may be purchased for educational, business, or sales promotional use. For information please write: Special Markets Department, HarperCollins Publishers, Inc., 10 East 53rd Street, New York, NY 10022.
FIRST EDITION

Designed by Nancy Singer

Library of Congress Cataloging-in-Publication Data

Hanson, Harry, 1961–
    Get your rear in gear : firming, toning, and shaping your butt / Harry Hanson with Robin K. Levinson. — 1st Harper perennial ed.
        p.   cm.
    ISBN 0-06-095140-0
    1. Exercise.   2. Buttocks.   I. Levinson, Robin K.   II. Title.
GV508.H35   1997   96-26044
613.7'1—dc20

96 97 98 99 00 ❖/RRD 10 9 8 7 6 5 4 3 2 1

CONTENTS

ACKNOWLEDGMENTS

Many people helped make this book a reality. I offer my thanks to:

Rich Henriksen, one of the personal trainers at Hanson Fitness System, who helped me come up with many of the exercises for this book;

Robin K. Levinson, an award-winning writer with outstanding interviewing and organizational skills, who accurately and enthusiastically translated my energy and philosophy into the written word;

Literary agents Angela Miller and Judith Riven, who brought Robin and me together and also provided support and guidance;

All the other clients at Hanson Fitness System who graciously contributed their opinions and insights;

Chiropractor Dr. Peter Plumb; certified massage therapist Joan Plumb; William E. Rovner, vice president for public affairs at HIP Health Plan of New Jersey; physical therapists Halas Basatemur, Ph.D., and Louise Plano, P.A., both of Central New Jersey Medical Group; and registered dietitian Helene Y. Dubin, M.S., for their guidance;

Marilyn Allan, copyright specialist at the American Heart Association National Center in Dallas, and Bruce Inverso of the American Heart Association's New Jersey affiliate, for their input and support.

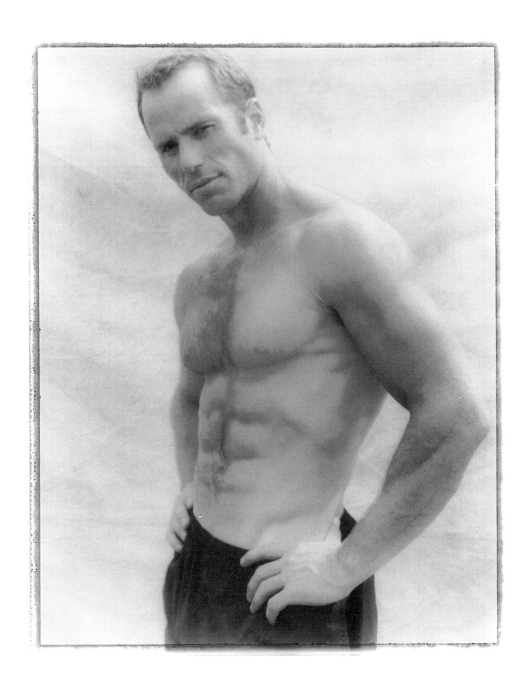

INTRODUCTION

"... Three, SQUEEZE IT. Two, SQUEEZE IT. One, SQUEEZE IT. Hold it, hold it, good. Isolate that muscle. Visualize it getting tighter. Can you feel it? Don't forget to breathe. Now ten more. Ten, SQUEEZE IT. Nine, SQUEEZE IT. Eight ... "

You are eavesdropping as I coach Debbie through a set of buttock lifts, one of a series of exercises designed to tone up and slim down her rear end. Like hundreds of people I've trained over the past decade, Debbie has been frustrated by her inability to change the shape and size of her hips and rear end. Like you who have opened this book, Debbie has come to me for help.

I'm Harry Hanson, competitive power lifter, personal trainer, and developer of the Hanson Fitness System here at Hanson's Gym in the SoHo district of Manhattan. What is the Hanson Fitness System? It is a simple, straightforward, yet highly effective exercise, diet, and motivational program I have designed to help Debbie and you get your rear—and the rest of your body—in gear.

As a personal trainer, I'm a fitness expert who educates and motivates you to exercise safely, productively, and frequently enough so you will lose fat, strengthen your muscles, and "sculpt" your way to a leaner, healthier, and more attractive body. This book is my opportunity to become *your* personal trainer. In my gym, it is the goal of each trainer to educate, motivate, and dictate the workout for our clients. And that's exactly what I'll do in the pages of *Get Your Rear in Gear*.

I have personally trained celebrities such as Demi Moore, Tom Cruise, Julia Roberts, Woody Harrelson, John F. Kennedy Jr., Kevin Anderson, D. B. Sweeney, Isaac Mizrahi, Ron Greshner, Mark Goodman, Meg Foster, Vincent Spano, Ron Rifkin, Fisher Stevens, Michael Cerveris, and Robin Morris. I've also trained models Naomi Campbell, Tyra Banks, Mary Mize, Crissa Anderson, Kim Warren, Megan Douglas, and Linda Evangelista—women whose very livelihoods depend on the shapeliness of their bodies. But by and large, our clients are just regular folks—hardworking, busy people who have made a commitment to improve their appearance, self-confidence, strength, endurance, and health. We use the same low-key, down-to-earth, nonjudgmental approach for celebrities and noncelebrities alike. We strive to make the pain painless and the exercises user-friendly.

Just as I do with the clients in my gym, I will help you, through this book, set realistic long-term fitness goals for yourself. Then I will show you exactly how to attain your objectives through a series of short-term goals. Once you reach your long-term goals, I'll help you set new goals or create a maintenance program that you can stick with.

Lack of motivation to stick with an exercise program is a major reason why one-third of Americans are obese. If you are one of them or are otherwise unhappy with your rear end, regardless of whether you've exercised before, you've come to the right place. The Hanson Fitness System has inspired and motivated thousands of people to abandon their poor eating habits and sedentary lifestyles. Beginners in particular respond to my approach because I never resort to guilt trips or insults. I firmly believe that no one is too out of shape to make the necessary changes to improve his or her fitness and self-esteem.

It is my sincere hope that this book will motivate you to become your own cheerleader. Instead of putting yourself down for not exercising long enough or hard enough, I want you to look in the mirror and say, "Way to go!" after your exercise session, no matter how short it was. Even if you can do only five quarter-squats or walk just two blocks, remind yourself that this is more than you did yesterday. Peppered throughout this book are powerful tips designed to help you keep your long-term motivation level as high as possible.

Beginners also like my program because I realize that not everybody is seeking the perfect rear end or the perfect body. Most of the people who pick up this book would probably be satisfied with dropping a dress size or two or looking better in jeans. I want to help you work exercise into your life—not your life into exercise. Of course, if you aspire to look as good as a fashion model, the Hanson Fitness System can put you on that road, too.

I also know that your attitude toward exercise can change from week to week, day to day, even hour to hour. My program accounts for this by showing you how to structure each workout to meet your current needs. If you are not feeling so great one day, we'll focus the workout session on getting your blood moving. If your muscles are sore, we might concentrate on stretching. The key is to keep yourself motivated enough to stick with the program.

Over the years my clients have reaffirmed my confidence in the Hanson Fitness System: "Harry made me believe I could do it," says John, a forty-two-year-old publishing executive. "I used to get to the seventh rep [repetition] and feel tired. Harry tells you you've got to keep going. He coaxes you through the last three reps until you're not only disciplined but hooked on exercise."

"The exercises have definitely changed the shape of my rear end; it looks like it's going up," says thirty-one-year-old Allison, an advertising producer who has been using the Hanson Fitness System off and on for five years.

Clara, fifty-six, an art researcher and consultant who went from a size eight to a size six in eighteen months, has made similar progress. "The exercises have made a remarkable difference, especially in my upper thighs and hips," Clara says. "I was never able to wear pants before. I even look better in bathing suits." As an added benefit, the exercises have led to an increase in Clara's bone density—a factor that can ward off osteoporosis, a debilitating, bone-thinning condition that runs in her family.

I, too, have made significant changes in my appearance thanks to the Hanson System. Over the course of six months in 1993, I went from 238 pounds to 190. I've kept those forty-eight pounds off ever since. How did I do it? The key word here is *gradually*. I didn't merely make a New Year's resolution and then radically turn my lifestyle around the next day. I had tried that tack before and always failed.

At the beginning of November 1992, I began preparing myself both emotionally and intellectually to improve my eating and exercise habits. For eight weeks, I psyched myself up, read up on nutrition, and tried some fat-free recipes. I scouted out local restaurants that had a variety of low-fat and fat-free menu items. As I became more acutely aware of my bad habits, I began to feel guilty whenever I ate something that was bad for me or skipped an exercise session because I was too tired or busy. Just as when you prepare for a long vacation or career change, I needed this time to ready myself for a new exercise and diet program in order to raise my chances of success.

Then, on New Year's Day 1993, I began gradually to increase the frequency of my workouts. I went from three days a week to four, five, six, and eventually seven. Whenever I planned out my week, I made sure I scheduled at least thirty minutes a day for exercise. Today, I run on a treadmill or do some other cardiovascular work for forty-five minutes a day. In addition, I do at least twenty minutes of strength-training exercises three or four times a week. This may seem like a lot, but my workouts account for just a small percentage of my total waking hours.

A couple of weeks after stepping up exercise, I began gradually to reduce my fat intake. Within a couple of months, I was consuming no more than fifteen grams of fat per day, which is low for the average person. My main approach was to stop adding butter, oil, and other forms of fat to my food; my research revealed that most foods, even bread, already have some fat in them, and I decided that all that extra fat just wasn't necessary. And I was right—now I don't even miss it. I also started reducing the size of my portions.

As I began shedding fat and looking and feeling better, my motivation to continue this new lifestyle increased. Now, my craving for fatty foods is virtually nonexistent. As I write this, there are probably three pumpkin pies in my refrigerator—and I am not the least bit tempted to taste them. At restaurants, my wife may order fried foods and dessert, but I have no desire for even a forkful. The idea of eating such things no longer enters my mind.

I maintain my diet and exercise plan with as much gusto as I put into playing with my daughter. You can do the same. Think about how much drive and intensity you have for your work, family, friends, or hobbies. Then transfer some of that intensity into your diet and exercise program. Everyone has the capacity to do this. It's simply a matter of tapping into your natural enthusiasm and redirecting it.

1

GETTING YOUR REAR
IN FIRST GEAR

A few years ago, *GQ* magazine asked me to survey my clients on which muscle group they thought could use the most improvement. After speaking with seventy or so clients, both male and female, as well as with several dozen friends, acquaintances, and family members, I found a general consensus that the part of the body that needed the most conditioning was the rear end. I wasn't surprised. Clothes hang better on the body when the rear is in shape. A well-formed rear also gives you more sex appeal. Remember the scene from the 1993 movie *Sleepless in Seattle* when widowed father Sam Baldwin asks a buddy for advice on what women look for in a man? The answer: "Sex—and a cute butt."

Visual appeal aside, having a well-toned rear end helps support the whole body. Your biggest muscles are located in your rear end. Making them stronger will enable you to tackle stairs without getting fatigued. You will be able to lift heavy objects more easily. You will be able to walk, jog, or run farther and more effortlessly than you could when your rear was weak and flabby.

If the muscles of the rear are so large, why is the rear end such a difficult body part to train? One reason is that it is out of sight and thus difficult to visualize, even with a mirror. Because it is hard to see, it is easy to forget about when you are exercising. Unlike the biceps of the upper arm, which are easily observed hardening and enlarging with the slightest lift of a dumbbell, the muscles of the rear are covered with several layers of fat. This makes the muscle group difficult to isolate both mentally and physically. The Hanson Fitness System will help you develop a mind-body connection that will put you in touch with this problem area. The system emphasizes proper form, balance, and body mechanics, which will enable you to exercise your rear muscles as efficiently and effectively as possible.

WHO CAN BENEFIT FROM THE HANSON FITNESS SYSTEM?

My clientele has ranged from high school athletes to sedentary senior citizens. People of all ages and walks of life stick with my one-on-one personal training program because they find it challenging and fun and, more important, because they are thrilled with the results.

Like the individualized training offered at Hanson's Gym, *Get Your Rear in Gear* can be used by people at all fitness levels. But I wrote this book primarily with the beginner in mind. All sorts of people might fall into the "beginner" category: the person who has never exercised before and doesn't know where to start; the new mother who needs to shed excess weight gained during pregnancy; the formerly active person who wants to get back into shape; or the extraordinarily busy businessperson who can spare only twenty minutes three times a week for exercise.

Another target audience includes people who have been working out regularly at home or at a gym but who need more guidance and inspiration. They may be unsure about their form, they may not know which exercises will do the most for their rear end, or they may feel that their progress has slowed or stagnated. *Get Your Rear in Gear* will show them how to fight boredom and motivate themselves to work out when they are feeling lazy.

Most of the rear-end exercises, which appear in Chapters Six through Eight, can be done in the privacy of your home. One reason I take this approach is to encourage overweight people who may be intimidated or embarrassed by the idea of working out in the showy, competitive atmosphere of the typical gym or fitness center. If you want to lose some weight so you will feel comfortable joining a gym, this book can get you there. Even if you have no desire ever to work out alongside others, the

Hanson Fitness System can help you look like you are a regular at the local fitness center.

HOW BADLY DO YOU WANT TO CHANGE YOUR BODY?

Results from any fitness program greatly depend on the level of your desire for improvement. If you want to trim your rear end and get the rest of your body in shape, simply wishing it so won't be enough. Your desire to succeed must outweigh your fear of taking a risk and making a sacrifice. It's like anything else in life. If you want to start a business, you must be willing to risk money and sacrifice time with friends and family. If you want to quit smoking, you must give up a source of pleasure and endure withdrawal symptoms. If you want to succeed in a relationship, you must be able to put someone else's needs before your own and risk getting hurt. If you want to shape up, you must turn down tempting but fattening foods, dedicate time to exercise, and be willing to put up with some temporary pain and soreness to achieve your goal. Never let yourself forget that the rewards of being your own boss, being a nonsmoker, having a loving relationship, and getting your body into better condition—are enormously high.

TAPPING YOUR MOTIVATION

Every New Year's Day, millions of Americans resolve to get their bodies into better shape. They spend their hard-earned money on athletic shoes, jogging suits, exercise bikes, treadmills, health-club memberships, aerobic dance classes, and the like. Research has found, though, that after three months, about 50 percent of these people will have abandoned their exercise routines. Why do so many people slip back into their easy chairs?

"I wasn't seeing any results."
"I became bored."
"It hurt too much."
"I couldn't find enough time to exercise."
"I hated all that work and sweat."

"I got injured."

"It became too expensive."

The reasons vary from person to person. But lurking behind every ex-exerciser's excuse are three simple words: lack of motivation.

Scholars define motivation as thoughts and feelings that initiate or intensify behavior. Simply put, motivation is that "get-up-and-go" attitude, the ability to start something and stick with it no matter what gets in the way. When you are motivated to exercise, you can fight off laziness. You have the wherewithal to stick with your program of physical activity, even when you travel, even when your schedule is thrown off by events in other areas of life. You exercise for exercise's sake, for the sheer joy of pushing yourself to do your best. To you, exercise is not a means to an end but an end in and of itself.

For most of us, motivation comes easily in the beginning. We are energized by our resolve to look and feel better. What's difficult is maintaining our motivation over the long haul. People lose interest because they don't see immediate signs of progress. They may be having a hard time fitting exercise into their schedules. Or they don't know which specific exercises will help them achieve their personal objectives.

The fact that you've picked up this book indicates that you have made a conscious decision to improve your body and your health. Right now you are brimming with motivation and enthusiasm. Good for you. Part of my job is to teach you how to keep your motivation level high. Toward that end, I offer you an array of practical motivational tips, which are scattered throughout the pages of this book. Each tip is crafted to inspire you to keep the Hanson System exercise and diet plan in high gear from now on. After all, stationary bikes and Nordic Tracks are too expensive to be used as clothes racks.

The tips come from my own life, the experiences of my clients, the *Tufts University Diet and Nutrition Newsletter,* and from reports by researchers Rod K. Dishman, Ph.D., of the Department of Exercise Science at the University of Georgia, Athens, and Rebecca Lewthwaite of the Department of Human Kinetics at the University of Wisconsin, Milwaukee. The tips are geared toward exercise, but most can be adapted to the nutritional arena as well.

Not all tips will work for all people. Experiment. Find out what works for you, based on your personality and motivational history. If one method stops working after a while, try something new. Or be creative.

Combine two or more tips, or invent some of your own. If they work, they're valid.

THE HANSON FITNESS SYSTEM PHILOSOPHY

When I first opened my gym in the mid-1980s, I used technical terms and big words while coaching my clients through their exercise routines. My clients weren't impressed. I didn't need to keep proving to them that I knew what I was talking about. I finally realized that they just wanted to train hard and have a good time. So I simplified my terminology. Simplicity has since become the cornerstone of my approach.

Another important aspect of my philosophy is to avoid overtraining and pushing people too hard. If you push people beyond their ability or make them exercise too hard, they become nauseous, they burn out, or worse, they get injured. When I first went into business for myself, I worked one hundred hours a week, trained eighteen people a day, engaged in my own rigorous exercise routine, cleaned the gym after hours, and ate and went to the bathroom only when I absolutely had to. Eventually, this frenzied pace caused my body to break down. I needed two stomach operations. After that experience, I turned my life around.

Tip No. 1: Educate Yourself

●

You probably know that exercise makes muscles stronger and burns fat. But did you know that aerobic exercise may strengthen your immune system, which helps ward off colds and other illnesses? That devout exercisers have lower rates of adult-onset diabetes and certain cancers? That exercise may reduce your risk of heart attack and stroke by 40 percent or more? In addition, vigorous exercise, such as walking or running fifteen miles a week, appears to increase longevity.

Learning about all the wonderful things that exercise does for your inside may help shake off the frustrations you may feel when you can't see rapid improvements on your outside. Almost every day, newspapers and magazines publish articles touting the various health benefits of exercise. Saving these articles in a fitness scrapbook will not only advance your "physical education" but also will give you something to read whenever you need inspiration to throw out that doughnut, turn off the television, and take a walk.

Today, I work out hard but not to the point of exhaustion. I give my muscles time to rest and recover. I train clients only in the morning, leaving the afternoons free for paperwork, phone calls, and other business matters. And when I'm home with my wife and young daughter, I'm with them 100 percent.

A third aspect to my philosophy is to maintain a healthy respect for my clients. I've worked with many personal trainers over the years and found that many project a holier-than-thou attitude. This attitude can intimidate clients or turn them off to exercise. At Hanson Fitness, my employees set an example by keeping their own bodies well conditioned, but I won't tolerate any trainer acting as though he or she is better than someone else. I have fired employees on the spot for criticizing a client or becoming visibly frustrated when a client couldn't complete a set or do an exercise correctly. I want my clients, as well as the readers of this book, to know how much I appreciate and respect them and their efforts.

Hanson Fitness System trainers offer liberal doses of praise as clients complete a workout. We are quick to notice and point out improvements in their bodies. And when clients do an exercise improperly or have trouble sticking with their diet, we nudge them back onto the wagon in a gentle, positive, encouraging way. This book will show you how to do the same for yourself. The value of encouragement cannot be overestimated. Think of the last time your boss said, "Terrific job," or "Great suggestion." A good supervisor knows that praise, when warranted, motivates employees to work harder. Self-praise can do the same thing in the realm of work—or working out. Criticizing yourself or simply failing to acknowledge your accomplishments cultivates a bad attitude that can prevent you from doing your best.

Variety is another feature that makes the Hanson Fitness System successful. Many personal trainers take their clients through the same workout day after day. I believe in mixing up the workout, focusing on cardiovascular

---

Tip No. 2: Be Sure You Are Ready to Make a Change

If you've just moved, gotten divorced, or begun a new job, this may not be the best time to launch significant long-term lifestyle changes. Stress in other areas of your life may affect your ability to cope with the stress of permanently changing your level of physical activity. Consider waiting until the rest of your life is more in control before beginning your exercise program.

training one day and toning exercises the next, for example.

This book takes the same overall approach as I do when I train myself, and it's not overly intense. You don't have to train as though you were a marathon runner or a triathlete. You just need to follow some simple instructions. The instructions, by the way, are exactly the same for men and women. Although the natural shape of the male's rear end is quite different from that of the female's, the musculature is identical.

Tip No. 3: Don't View Exercise as Optional

———————●———————

Getting adequate exercise is just as important to your overall health as eating sensibly, getting enough sleep, and wearing your seat belt.

HOW THE SYSTEM WORKS

The Hanson Fitness System for getting your rear in gear takes a three-pronged approach. First is cardiovascular training, commonly known as aerobic exercise. The second approach is to cut some fat and calories from your diet. Third is the series of strength-training exercises described and illustrated in Chapters Six through Eight. Individually, exercise and nutritional modification are beneficial. But changes in your body will be quicker, more dramatic, more gratifying, and longer lasting when you combine all three.

Cardiovascular Fitness

Nature designed our rear end as a storehouse for fat. Fat layers help cushion our rears so we can sit down comfortably. Storing fat in the hips, buttocks, and thighs also makes sense because these areas are relatively distant from vital organs that can be damaged by too much fatty tissue. The downside is that the body burns excess fat from the hips and buttocks last rather than first, so to slim down the rear end, you must burn more fat in general. The only way to do this is to engage in some form of cardiovascular workout for twenty to forty-five minutes at least three times a week.

The kind of cardiovascular exercise you do is not as important as the frequency and intensity with which you do it. In Chapter Three, you'll find a chart to help you identify your fat-burning "training zone" heart rate; a companion chart lists the number of calories the average person burns during a variety of cardiovascular workouts. I will show you how easy it is to incorporate cardiovascular activities into your normal routine.

A word of caution: everyone—especially beginners, those with medical conditions including obesity, a history of heart or lung disease, or physical limitations, and anyone age forty-five or older—should get a doctor's approval before attempting the rear-end exercises or any cardiovascular workout. The questionnaire at the end of this chapter is designed to help you identify any potential risk factors you might have.

Nutritional Modification

Every year, Americans spend billions of dollars on diet programs. The Hanson Fitness System of nutritional modification costs next to nothing. The formula is simple: use the chart in Chapter Four to figure out how many calories you need to maintain your present weight. Keep a diary of how many calories you take in during a normal day. The next day, trim fifty or one hundred calories by reducing your portions. Gradually reduce your fat intake to 20 percent or less of total calories, and the pounds will start to melt off. Chapter Four offers more than two dozen tips that will painlessly and deliciously improve your eating habits. These tips include nibbling your way to a leaner body and looking in the mirror when you crave a Milky Way.

Tip No. 4: Work Exercise into Your Life

●

When you write out your weekly calendar, don't forget to schedule time to exercise. Write it down in pen, not pencil. Then jealously guard this "quality time" for your body.

If your life is extremely busy, consider waking up a half hour early to jog in place or do your rear-end exercises while you watch the morning news. This will work only if you are a "morning person." If you are an "afternoon person," bring a bag lunch to work and spend your lunch hour power-walking around the block. You can eat at your desk later. (Power-walking is walking as fast as you can without jogging; most people can power-walk one mile in fifteen minutes or less.)

If you have the greatest amount of energy in the evening, tell your family that dinner will be served a half hour later on certain days. Or delegate cooking duty to someone else, and exercise as soon as you get home. Another option is to eat a light dinner and exercise afterward.

Rear-End Toning Exercises

These are strength-training exercises designed to condition the muscles of the rear end: the gluteus maximus, the gluteus medius, and the gluteus minimus, collectively known as the "gluteals" or "glutes." These exercises will also indirectly tone other common trouble spots: the inner and outer thighs and, to a lesser degree, the abdomen and lower back. In Chapter Two, you will read about the gluteals and surrounding muscle groups in greater detail. You will also learn how and why muscles burn fat in order to contract. Understanding some of the intricacies of this amazing tissue will help you form that all-important mind-body connection: the ability to visualize and isolate your muscles as you exercise.

The exercise chapters are divided into three levels of difficulty: Chapter Six offers Stage One exercises, geared toward beginners. Chapter Seven contains Stage Two exercises for people at the intermediate fitness level. Stage Three exercises, the most challenging series, are found in Chapter Eight. Most of the Stage One exercises are known as "manual exercises" because they do not require access to gyms, free weights, or exercise machines. The few that require exercise machines are optional. If you exercise at home, you will need a mat or carpeted floor.

You will need a set of dumbbells for many of the intermediate and advanced exercises. Dumbbells are quite inexpensive and easy to store. There are also optional exercises that require exercise machines. As you progress to more difficult exercises, you may want to consider investing in

---

Tip No. 5: Be Patient

●

Some people stop exercising because they don't see results soon enough. They perceive exercise only as a means to an end, a chore they must endure in order to wear size eight jeans. If after two months of exercising two or three times a week, they haven't lost a significant number of pounds or inches, they throw up their hands and quit. "We're all into this immediate-gratification thing," one of my clients, thirty-three-year-old Madeleine Gold, points out. "It gives us an excuse to give up if we don't see immediate changes after two months. . . . You have to realize it may take one or two years. You can't make yourself nuts looking in the mirror every day thinking, 'My butt hasn't changed.'"

Even if you exercise for an hour every day, progress may still be gradual. Everyone loses weight at different rates: some take pounds off quickly; others take a while. Indeed, losing weight slowly—no more than a pound a week—has been shown to be healthier and longer lasting than rapid weight loss.

home exercise equipment or joining a gym. My recommendations on exercise machines appear in Chapter Five. Another option is to concentrate only on the manual exercises but use heavier free weights and increase your reps. To determine your current fitness level, take the quiz in Chapter Five.

This book offers almost sixty rear-end exercises: twenty-four Stage One, eighteen Stage Two, and seventeen Stage Three. I offer many choices, not so you will feel compelled to do them all during any given workout but so you will be able to vary your workout with ease. Doing different exercise combinations trains your rear end and surrounding muscle groups from different angles, and it also helps you fight boredom.

Photographs coupled with clear, concise descriptions in all three exercise chapters will show you how to use correct form. In addition to preventing injuries, correct form is crucial to the effectiveness of any exercise. If your form is off while doing a squat, for example, you might waste energy working other muscle groups that you may not want to make bigger. That energy is best channeled into squeezing your rear-end muscles. Far worse, improper form can lead to knee or back injuries or undue muscle soreness. Injury and unnecessary pain are common reasons why people give up on exercise.

HOW TO MAKE THIS BOOK WORK FOR YOU

If you are just starting out on a fitness program, I urge you to read all the chapters before trying any rear-end exercises. This way, you will under-

---

Tip No. 6: Keep Your Expectations Realistic

Unless you have a genetic predisposition to be incredibly thin and flawlessly beautiful, don't compare yourself to professional models like Naomi Campbell and Linda Evangelista. These are women in their twenties who were born beautiful and have a very slender natural body structure. Unfortunately, we live in a society that defines beauty as weighing 105 pounds and being five feet ten inches tall. Don't buy into this mind-set; having a supermodel's physique is neither healthy nor attainable for the vast majority of people. In most cases, expecting that exercise will result in a body that movie stars would envy sets you up for disappointment and exercise burnout.

While you shouldn't expect immediate changes in your appearance, it is reasonable to expect to feel better psychologically just a few days or weeks after beginning your fitness program. Getting involved in exercise will give you a better outlook and make you feel better about yourself. Many of my clients report feeling more in control of their lives, less stressed, and more mentally focused after exercising. Says one of my clients, Deborah Friedman, an art dealer from New York, "If something is bothering me, something I might go to a therapist to talk about, I find that physical exercise helps me deal with it. . . . If I don't think about my problem and just exercise, somehow it all works out."

stand how all the system's components fit together. I'll also bet that after reading through the book, you will be motivated—perhaps more than ever before in your life—to make a long-term commitment to getting your body in shape and keeping it that way.

If you are already in decent condition—if you exercise regularly and watch your diet—you can go directly to the intermediate or advanced strength-training exercises. Chapters Two through Five will, however, serve as refreshers for you; you may even learn something new or discover a different twist on what you are already doing.

STATE YOUR OBJECTIVES

Before you continue, please fill out the following questionnaire, which is designed to help you crystallize your goals and anticipate potential obstacles. You may need to update your answers from time to time.

THE HANSON FITNESS SYSTEM
QUESTIONNAIRE

1. What are your objectives for participating in the Hanson Fitness System of exercise training and nutritional modification?

_____

_____

_____

_____

2. What aspects of your rear end would you like to change?

_____

_____

_____

_____

3. What, if anything, in the past has held you back from improving your level of physical fitness?

_____

_____

_____

_____

4. What, if anything, might interfere with your ability to exercise at least three times a week?

_____

_____

_____

_____

5. MEDICAL HISTORY. Describe any past or current sports- or exercise-related injuries or problems you have had, including muscle pulls, sprains, fractures, surgery, chronic pain, or any general discomfort.

HEAD/NECK:

_____

_____

SHOULDER/CLAVICLE:

_____

_____

ARM/ELBOW/WRIST/HAND:

_____

_____

BACK:

_____

_____

HIP/PELVIS:

_____

_____

THIGH/KNEE:

_____

_____

LOWER LEG/ANKLE/FOOT:

_____

_____

(If you filled out any part of question 5, show this questionnaire and the exercises in Chapters Six through Eight to your family physician, sports medicine doctor, exercise physiologist, or physical therapist. A medical professional should be able to tell you which, if any, rear-end exercises to avoid.)

6. HEART/LUNG RISK FACTORS. Please answer yes (Y) or no (N) to the following:

( ) Do you smoke?

( ) Have you stopped smoking in the past year?

( ) Has anyone in your family (your parents, grandparents, brothers, sisters, children) ever suffered a heart attack?

( ) Has anyone in your family ever suffered a heart attack before age forty-five?

( ) Does anyone in your family have diabetes that began during adulthood?

( ) Does anyone in your family have high blood pressure?

( ) Have you ever had an abnormal electrocardiogram?

( ) Have you ever had an abnormal exercise stress test finding?

(If you answered yes to any of these questions, get a doctor's approval before embarking on this or any other exercise program.)

7. Check the boxes corresponding to diseases or conditions that your physician has diagnosed or treated you for. Include past and present conditions.

( ) Diabetes

( ) Hypoglycemia

( ) Frequent skin infections, acne, or recurrent boils

( ) High blood cholesterol

( ) High blood triglycerides

( ) High blood pressure

( ) Prior heart attack or chest pains (angina)

( ) Gout

( ) Rheumatoid arthritis

( ) Osteoarthritis

( ) More than three colds a year

( ) Chronic constipation

( ) Irritable bowel syndrome

( ) Diverticulosis or diverticulitis

( ) Nervousness or excessive anxiety

( ) Frequent insomnia

( ) Hiatal hernia

( ) Stomach ulcers

( ) Fibrocystic breast disease

( ) Iron-deficiency anemia

( ) Sickle cell anemia

( ) Frequent or chronic canker sores in the mouth (not herpes)

( ) Chronic or frequent leg ulcers due to circulatory problems

( ) Recurrent genital herpes

( ) Recurrent oral herpes

( ) Excessive perspiration odor

( ) Poor sense of taste or smell

( ) Asthma triggered by exercise

( ) Recurrent attacks of phlebitis

( ) Cirrhosis of the liver

( ) Congestive heart failure

( ) Claudication of the legs (Do you walk with a limp?)

( ) Kidney failure requiring dialysis

( ) Lactose intolerance (inability to digest milk sugars)

(If you checked any of these items, get a physician's approval before starting the program described in this book.)

YOUR RESPONSIBILITY

This book tells you exactly what you must do to get your rear end in shape and improve your overall level of fitness. I give you the formula as simply as I can. How far you want to take it is up to you.

Tip No. 8: Set Attainable Goals

Keep your short-term goals modest. For instance, add one minute to your cardiovascular workout. Walk a block more than you did last week. Increase repetitions of your rear-end exercises by one.

Long-term goals should also be realistic and as simple as possible. How specific they are will vary from person to person. "I want to improve my overall fitness level," "I want to climb the stairs without getting winded," or "I want to wear the clothes that have been hanging in my closet for five years" are perfectly acceptable and attainable long-term goals. If your long-term goal is more formidable, such as shedding thirty pounds or more, break it down. Set your first long-term goal at losing ten pounds. Once you've done that, shoot for dropping ten more. By keeping long-term goals incremental, you'll experience more successes. A taste of success almost always inspires you to reach for more.

While it certainly helps to set goals, don't overstate their importance. Exercise has intrinsic value; it is more than a path toward looking better in a bathing suit.

2

MUSCLES:
THE GEARS OF THE REAR

Muscle is nature's most perfect engine. It is made to move. If a muscle goes too long without moving, it atrophies—that is, it becomes smaller and weaker. With movement, muscles stay toned, and with regular exercise, muscles gets bigger, stronger, and more flexible. Strong muscles help protect our bones and improve our posture, and they burn fat faster and more efficiently. Even at rest, strong muscles use more calories per minute than poorly conditioned muscles. Later in this chapter you will find out why. But first, let's put them in perspective.

TYPES OF MUSCLE

The human body has three varieties of muscle tissue: the cardiac muscle of the heart, the smooth muscles of the digestive tract and other internal organs, and the skeletal muscles, which are responsible for moving the joints of the skeleton. Cardiac and smooth muscles are considered "involuntary" because they function automatically without our having to think about them. Skeletal muscles are called "voluntary muscles" because we can move them at will. We have more than 650 individual voluntary muscles, most of which are bundled into muscle groups. Each muscle is attached to bone or to other muscles by extremely strong fibrous cords called tendons.

The single largest muscle in the human body is the gluteus maximus—the rear end. Together with two smaller rear-end muscles, the gluteus medius and gluteus minimus, the gluteus maximus enables us to sit down, stand up, walk, jog, run, dance, kick, climb, skip, hop, ski, and engage in many other physical activities. Sprinters, speed skaters, and power lifters develop rock-hard rear-end muscles, or "gluteals," in order to excel at their respective sports. Nonathletes covet firm gluteals as a means of looking better and feeling stronger.

To help you achieve these goals, in this book I offer rear-end exercises that focus primarily on the gluteus maximus, medius, and minimus. The type and extent of changes you would like to see in your rear end determine which exercises you do and how hard you train. If you want the upper part of your rear end to rise higher on your torso, for example, concentrate on the exercises that isolate the gluteus medius. If you want to bring out the roundness of your rear, isolate the gluteus maximus. If your rear end is sagging or a little droopy, you'll want to train the minimus and the maximus simultaneously. By doing the exercises in Chapters Six through Eight, you will challenge to a lesser degree your thigh and abdominal muscles, and you will indirectly tone the major muscles in your back. Descriptions of each exercise will tell you which of the following muscles it trains, either directly or indirectly.

MUSCLES OF THE REAR

Gluteus Maximus

Although you might think your rear end is composed primarily of fat, you can actually change the fat-to-muscle ratio so that your rear end is mostly muscle. The bulk of that muscle tissue is the gluteus maximus, a wide, thick muscle that wraps around the exterior of hips and buttocks. It extends from the hipbone and the bones at the base of the spine around to the upper portion of thighbone. Its major movements are extending the leg backward and rotating the pelvis and thighs. The massive gluteus maximus is one of the body's strongest muscles.

Gluteus Medius

Situated just beneath the lower half of the gluteus maximus, the gluteus medius is a smaller muscle that works to raise your leg out sideways. It also helps you balance your hips while walking or running.

Gluteus Minimus

This muscle lies under the upper portion of the gluteus maximus. It contracts in concert with the gluteus medius, performing the same basic movements.

MUSCLES OF THE THIGH

Sartorius

Our longest muscle, the sartorius, begins in the hip, runs along the inner thigh, and attaches to the back of the knee. Its main function is to rotate the thigh outward.

Tip No. 10: Dress for Success

When you are working out, the last thing you need is underwear that pinches or sneakers that give you blisters. When it comes to workout garb, make comfort your first consideration. Most of my clients wear shorts with elasticized waistbands and baggy T-shirts. If you feel comfortable in Spandex, by all means indulge yourself.

When I exercise alone at home, I sometimes turn up the thermostat and strip down to my underwear. Try it, if you feel comfortable. By exercising with little or no clothing in front of a mirror, you can watch your muscles contract, which will help foster a mind-body connection. (This will also motivate you to eat better.)

Adductors

This muscle group includes the adductor longus and the adductor magnus and runs from the pubic bone to the thighbone. Adductor muscles work with the sartorius to rotate and flex the legs and to pull the legs inward. The gracilis, a smaller muscle of the inner thigh, is also used in these movements.

Quadriceps

Whenever you straighten out a bent knee, you are using your quadriceps, a four-headed muscle located in the front of the thigh. The quadriceps includes three vastus muscles: the vastus lateralis, the vastus medialis, and the vastus intermedius. These three quadriceps "heads" originate at different points along the thighbone and terminate in the knee. The fourth head, the rectus femoris, begins at the front of the hipbone and also ends in the knee.

Tensor Fasciae Latae

This muscle runs along the outer thigh and contracts to lift the leg outward to the side.

Hamstrings

The back of the thigh is composed of three muscles known collectively as the hamstrings: the biceps femoris, the semimembranosus, and the semitendinosus. All three muscles begin in the pelvis and insert in the back of the knee. When hamstrings contract, the knee bends.

MUSCLES OF THE ABDOMEN

Rectus Abdominis

Bodybuilders and other serious athletes have a "rippling" abdomen that appears segmented like a washboard. This is the result of a highly conditioned rectus abdominis. The rectus abdominis is a broad, flat muscle that originates on the pubic bone, spans the abdominal region like a bridge, and inserts in the ribs parallel to the sternum and the two ribs just below it. Every few inches along the length of the rectus abdominis is a layer of connective tissue running horizontally. This unique segmentation evolved to support the bridge section of the muscle and to keep its length relatively constant. The rectus abdominis is the main engine when you are doing sit-ups.

External Obliques

Whenever you flex or twist your torso, you do it with the help of external obliques. These muscles, which form the waist, run diagonally from the rectus abdominis to the outside of the lower rib cage.

Tip No. 12: Do Something You Enjoy

Since your heart doesn't know or care whether you are swimming or playing racquetball, you might as well pursue a cardiovascular workout that you enjoy and are good at. If you are new to the exercise game, you may have to fish around for a while before finding an activity that is a good fit. If you enjoyed basketball in high school, find out if the local YMCA has a team you can join, or organize one yourself at work. If you took jazz dance or ballet lessons when you were young, you'd probably enjoy Jazzercise or another form of aerobic dance. If you are competitive by nature, try a racquet sport. If you love the outdoors, find a nice park with jogging trails. If you were born to shop, find out whether your local indoor shopping mall opens to walkers before business hours; not only will you get to walk year-round, you will make new friends and beat everyone to the sales when the stores open.

MUSCLES OF THE BACK

Latissimus Dorsi

This muscle spreads like a fan from the armpit over the back of the rib cage before ending along the spine. Its jobs include arching the lower back, twisting the torso, and straightening up after bending at the waist.

THE INNER LIFE OF THE MUSCLE

Muscles have one mission—to contract, or shorten—and they do it extraordinarily well. The striation, or stripes, that appear on the surface of skeletal muscles are the result of contraction chemistry.

Unlike the familiar round red blood cell, a muscle cell is a long, thin cylinder with several nuclei and at least one nerve ending. Because of their structure, muscle cells are commonly referred to as muscle fibers. Some muscle cells are a foot long.

Each muscle fiber contains several hundred or several thousand smaller fibers known as myofibrils. The configuration is similar to a telephone cable encasing many thin wires. Each myofibril contains countless filaments running parallel to one another. Filaments are made of proteins—long molecules of amino acids and other constituents. The thickness and thus the color of each filament are determined by the filament's protein. Darker, thicker filaments are made of a protein called myosin; lighter, thinner filaments are made up of the protein actin.

Sets of filaments are divided by thin membranes into numerous sections, or sarcomeres. Sarcomeres, the basic units of contraction, contain alternating filaments of dark myosin and light actin. This repeating pattern of light and dark zones is the source of striation.

Except in the case of a reflex, contraction of the striated muscles is initiated when the brain sends a signal through the spinal column to the striated

---

Tip No. 13: Use Mental Distractions

Working out on aerobic exercise equipment can be boring. But if you focus your mind on something else, the time will melt away as quickly as the fat. Listen to music, preferably something with a strong beat. Or watch something interesting on television. Or carry on a conversation with the person on the neighboring treadmill or stationary bike.

muscle fibers. When the order to contract is received, the myosin and actin filaments contract, shortening the myofibrils (the individual muscle fibers) and ultimately the muscle as a whole.

Fueling the Engines

In order to contract, muscle cells must burn fuel in the form of sugar or fatty acid (fat). At first, sugar in the form of glycogen is burned because it is stored in muscle tissue and thus is instantly available to the muscle cells. But glycogen is the only fuel that the brain and nerves can use. So to conserve glycogen, muscles consume it only to initiate activity, leaving the rest for the nervous system. Muscles start using fat as their primary fuel source as soon as the breathing and heart rate increase enough to bring more oxygen to the muscle cells. This changeover occurs several minutes after beginning a cardiovascular (aerobic) workout. Although the rear-end exercises are not aerobic per se, they can prompt muscles to burn more fat if you do your repetitions with as much speed and intensity as you can. More important, the exercises will promote muscle growth. The bigger your muscles are, the faster your resting metabolism will be—and the more calories you'll burn each day.

Tip No. 14: Get an Exercise Buddy

●

It is difficult to blow off your workout if someone is waiting for you at the gym or park. Having a buddy to exercise with also fights boredom and may add a sense of friendly competition.

Tip No. 15: Seek Outside Support

●

Let all your significant others know that you have made exercise a priority in your life. This way, they won't try to persuade you to do something else when you are planning to work out. This also generates a booster squad. You will have lots of people to brag to when you build up to a two-mile run or graduate to Stage Two exercises. As your friends and relatives see changes in your attitude and appearance, it may inspire them to join you in your fitness regimen.

The Engine's "Exhaust"

Like a car engine's exhaust, a contracting muscle produces by-products: heat, water, carbon dioxide, and a weak acid known as lactic acid. During exercise, heat is dissipated through sweating, and carbon dioxide is carried away by the circulatory system. Some of the lactic acid is converted to pyruvic acid, which muscle cells use to generate more energy. Lactic acid can also be made into glycogen by the muscles and the liver.

As exercise becomes more strenuous, a local buildup of lactic acid can occur. This is the source of muscle fatigue. You will know immediately when your muscles are fatigued because you will feel a burning sensation or the sharp pain of a muscle cramp. When a muscle cramps or the burn grows too intense to bear, stop exercising. Gently stretch or shake out the affected muscle to increase circulation through the area. This brings in additional oxygen and helps remove the excess lactic acid. As soon as the pain subsides, you can resume exercising.

Tip No. 16: Vary Your Workout

●

There are enough rear-end exercises in Chapters Six, Seven, and Eight that you can mix and match different ones during each workout session. When it is time for cardiovascular training, do more than one activity. For example, you can power-walk for ten or fifteen minutes, then bicycle for another ten or fifteen minutes. In a gym, you can spend five or ten minutes each on three different exercise machines, and skip rope for another five minutes. Or you can swim laps on Thursday, take an aerobics class on Friday, and go hiking over the weekend. Doing different activities in different surroundings prevents boredom and burnout. Varying your workouts also helps develop different muscle groups.

3

PUTTING HEART INTO YOUR WORKOUT

Knowing the importance of cardiovascular training, Larry wanted to combine physical fitness with his commute to work. So he threw a change of clothes into his backpack and bicycled the full twelve miles. After biking to work twice, however, he found himself dreading having to do it again. For one thing, he needed to drag himself out of bed before dawn in order to make it to his desk by 7:00 A.M. And he didn't get home until after dark.

As a compromise, Larry now puts his bike on a car rack and drives halfway to work. He parks in a shopping center parking lot and cycles the rest of the way, a little over six miles. His drive-bike commute, which he does two or three times a week depending on the weather, enables Larry to sleep in a little longer and to get home at a reasonable hour. Since his employer provides showers, Larry keeps soap, towels, and clean clothes in his desk.

Larry found a creative solution to working cardiovascular exercise into his life. This chapter will help you do the same.

As you will learn in Chapter Five, "Training Technique," there is only one correct way to do strength-training exercises like the ones in this book. When it comes to cardiovascular workouts, however, the type of exercise you do isn't as important as the fact that you do it.

To get the most out of your cardiovascular workout, your heart should beat within 50 percent to 75 percent of its maximum rate—this is your target zone. To estimate your maximum rate, subtract your age from 220. To find your target heart rate zone, look for the age category closest to your age in Chart 3.1 and read the line across. For example, if you are thirty, your target zone is 95 to 142 beats per minute. If you are forty-three, use the figures for age forty-five, the closest age on the chart. The numbers are the same for women and men.

Chart 3.1

●

FINDING YOUR TARGET HEART RATE (HR) ZONE

AGE	TARGET HR ZONE 50–75%	AVERAGE MAXIMUM Heart Rate 100%
20	100–150 beats per min.	200
25	98–146 beats per min.	195
30	95–142 beats per min.	190
35	93–138 beats per min.	185
40	90–135 beats per min.	180
45	88–131 beats per min.	175
50	85–127 beats per min.	170
55	83–123 beats per min.	165
60	80–120 beats per min.	160
65	78–116 beats per min.	155
70	75–113 beats per min.	150

Your maximum heart rate is approximately 220 minus your age. However, the figures in the chart are averages and should be used as general guidelines.

Note: A few high-blood-pressure medications lower the maximum heart rate and thus the target zone rate. If you are taking medication for high blood pressure, call your physician to find out if your exercise program needs to be adjusted.

(Reproduced with permission. Exercise and Your Heart: A Guide to Physical Activity, *copyright © 1993 American Heart Association.)*

To find your pulse, place your index or middle finger lightly on your inner wrist under your thumb or on your carotid artery, located on the side of your neck just beneath your jawbone. (Don't take your pulse with your thumb because your thumb has its own pulse.) When you feel the blood pulsing, look at your watch and count the number of pulses for ten seconds. Multiply that figure by six to get your heart rate per minute.

Take your pulse immediately after you stop exercising. If you are a beginner, pause to monitor your heart rate periodically during your workout to make sure your heart is not beating too rapidly. The heavier and more out of shape you are, the quicker your pulse will reach your target zone and the easier it will be for it to exceed that zone. As you lose weight and strengthen your heart through exercise, it will take longer to reach your target zone, and your heart rate will return to normal more quickly after you stop exercising.

Try to get some kind of cardiovascular workout at least three times a week. Start slowly so that your heart rate climbs to its training zone gradually. If you like, stop momentarily once you have broken a sweat to stretch your muscles gently. Here is a good stretching routine that hits all the body's major muscle groups. You can do these stretches before or after warming up, but be especially gentle if your muscles feel tight:

1: Stretch your arms out to your sides and do small clockwise circles for thirty to forty-five seconds. Then reach to the sky and out to your sides again and do counterclockwise circles for another thirty to forty-five seconds. This increases blood flow to your shoulder area.

2: Without turning your head, gently tilt your head from side to side three times and front and back three times. This increases flexibility in your neck area, a common injury site.

3: Bend over at the waist with your head down and try to touch your hands to the floor, your ankles, or your knees. Keeping your knees slightly bent, hang there for thirty to forty-five seconds. Don't bounce—bouncing can result in a pulled muscle if you are not warmed up. This bent-over stretch lengthens your lower back muscles and the muscles down the back of your legs. Round up out of the stretch very slowly, straightening up one vertebra at a time.

4: Placing your left hand on a wall for balance, bend your right knee, lifting your right foot up toward your rear. Grab your inner ankle with your right hand and pull your foot out behind you. Hold it for thirty seconds. Repeat with your other foot. This stretches your quadriceps (the front of your thighs).

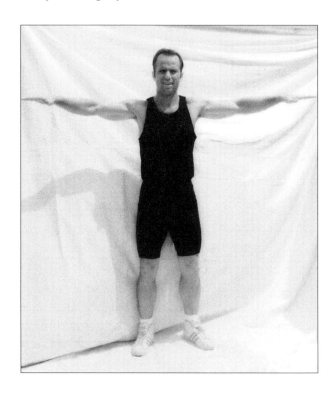

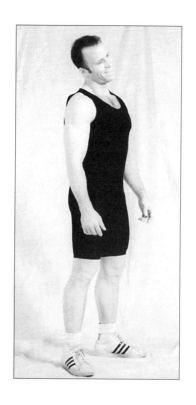

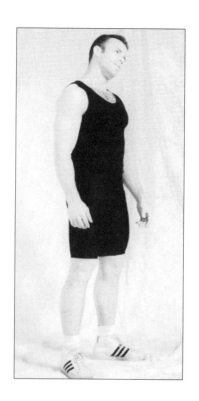

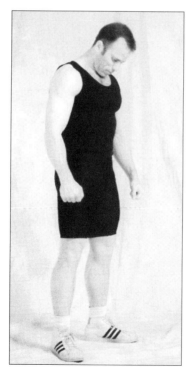

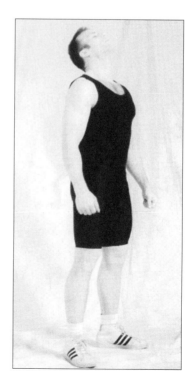

After stretching, start your cardiovascular exercise and continue until your heart rate has been in your target zone for at least twenty minutes. Then give yourself a cool-down period of about five minutes to allow your heartbeat to gradually return to its resting rate, which for most people ranges from 60 to 100 beats per minute. Cooling down also helps prevent muscle cramps. To cool down, continue the same exercise you have been doing but at a more leisurely pace. If your workout takes the form of tennis, soccer, or another demanding sport, walk around for five minutes after the game has ended. Once your heart rate has returned to normal, repeat the stretches just described. You'll probably notice that you are more flexible after your workout than before. You'll also notice after several months of regular cardiovascular workouts that your resting pulse has slowed down. This means your heart is getting stronger. Use Chart 3.2 to help you document your progress.

MAXIMIZING YOUR CARDIOVASCULAR WORKOUT

The following paragraphs suggest some more ways to make the most of your cardiovascular workout.

Don't Get Breathless

Always exercise at a comfortable pace. Don't let yourself get so winded that you cannot carry on a conversation. If it takes more than ten minutes after you stop exercising for your heart rate to return to normal, you may have exercised too vigorously for your fitness level. Other signs that you are exercising too vigorously include breathing with difficulty, feeling faint, and prolonged weakness during or after exercising, according to the American Heart Association.

Relax

Next time you are engaged in cardiovascular exercise, notice whether your hands are curled into fists, your jaw is clenched, or your lips are pursed. If any of these things is happening, you are wasting energy. When bicycling, for example, do not grip the bicycle handles too tightly. When walking or jogging, let your hands hang loosely and keep your lips and jaw relaxed.

Chart 3.2

CARDIOVASCULAR EXERCISE LOG

Week No._____

Dates_____**to**_____

Day	Activity	Heart Rate	How Far/ How Long
Sun.			
Mon.			
Tues.			
Wed.			
Thurs.			
Fri.			
Sat.			

Increase the Intensity

You can increase the intensity of any cardiovascular training session by going a little faster or exercising a bit longer. Wearing fins in the swimming pool, for example, will increase the resistance every time you kick, giving your legs a better workout. There are also training paddles for swimmers to wear on their hands.

Chart 3.3

●

CALORIES BURNED DURING SELECTED ACTIVITIES

The average calories spent per hour by a 150-pound person are listed below. (A lighter person burns fewer calories; a heavier person burns more.) Since exact calorie figures are not available for most activities, the figures below are averaged from several sources and show the relative vigor of the activities.

Activity	Calories/Hour
Bicycling (6 mph)	240
Bicycling (12 mph)	410
Cross-country skiing	700
Jogging (5½ mph)	740
Jogging (7 mph)	920
Jumping rope	750
Running in place	650
Running 10 mph	1,280
Swimming (25 yds./min.)	275
Swimming (50 yds./min.)	500
Tennis (singles)	400
Walking (2 mph)	240
Walking (3 mph)	320
Walking (4½ mph)	440

The calories spent in a particular activity vary in proportion to one's body weight. For example, a 100-pound person burns one-third fewer calories, so you would multiply the number of calories in the above chart by 0.7. For a 200-pound person, multiply by 1.3.

(Reproduced with permission. Exercise and Your Heart: A Guide to Physical Activity, *copyright © 1993 American Heart Association.)*

When walking, jogging, or bicycling outdoors, find some uphill grades to challenge yourself. Many stationary bicycles and treadmills can be adjusted to represent hills and valleys. If you want to target your rear-end muscles while bicycling, lean forward and use your whole foot and leg to pump while you mentally isolate your rear-end muscles. Standing up and pedaling also challenges the rear. Isolate different leg muscles by shifting your feet on the pedals. Push from your toes to hit the lower quadriceps; push from the heel to challenge your hamstrings; turn your feet slightly outward to isolate the muscles of the inner thigh.

Breathe Easy

Instead of breathing through your nose, inhale and exhale through your mouth during your cardiovascular workout. Nasal passages are much smaller than your trachea, which means you can deliver more oxygen to your muscles through mouth breathing, also known as "free-form breathing."

Break a Sweat

If you have been doing some form of cardiovascular exercise for ten minutes but are not sweating, you probably have not reached your target heart rate zone, and you are not burning fat. Step up your pace or increase the resistance.

Dash Training

An effective technique that can be used in any cardiovascular workout setting is "dash training." Dash training means alternating between working hard for as long as you can and easing up for a short while to catch your breath. In the case of bicycling, dash training can mean pedaling hard nonstop for a half mile, pedaling less strenuously and coasting for a quarter mile, then pedaling hard again. On a treadmill, dash training can mean walking for two minutes and power-walking for the next two, or switching back and forth from walking to jogging or sprinting.

For beginners, dash training is inviting because you can treat yourself to several "rest" periods even as you continue to burn calories. After a few weeks of dash training, you will find it easier to lengthen your intervals of high-intensity exercise and shorten your periods of low-intensity exercise. You should feel good about the progress you have made; even before you begin to lose weight, your heart is getting stronger and your overall level of fitness is improving. In a few months, if you keep at it, your need to ease up during your cardiovascular workout may even disappear.

PEPPING UP YOUR LIFESTYLE

There are other physical activities you can easily incorporate into your daily routine to burn some extra calories. Walk or jog in place during TV commercials, for example. Squeeze your rear end as tightly as you can while waiting for the bus or standing on line. Find a physically taxing hobby such as gardening. If you do not own a dog, offer to walk your neighbor's. Turn on music at home and dance, dance, dance. Playing actively with children can also help improve your fitness level and burn fat. Here are a few more suggestions[1]:

- Use the stairs—up and down—instead of the elevator. Start with one flight of stairs and gradually build up to more.
- Park a few blocks from the office or store and walk the rest of the way. Or if you ride on public transportation, get off a stop or two early and walk a few blocks.
- Take an activity break—get up and stretch, walk around, and give your muscles and mind a chance to relax.
- Instead of eating that extra snack, take a brisk stroll around the neighborhood.
- Do housework, such as vacuuming, at a brisker pace.
- Mow your own lawn.
- Go dancing instead of seeing a movie.
- Talk a walk after dinner instead of watching TV.

[1]*Reproduced with permission.* Exercise and Your Heart: A Guide to Physical Activity, *copyright © 1993 American Heart Association.*

4

DON'T GET BEAT BY WHAT YOU EAT

Over the last few decades, scientists have conducted a dizzying assortment of studies looking at the role that diet plays in weight loss. In my view, the researchers' often confusing and sometimes conflicting conclusions can be boiled down to this: reduce your calorie and fat consumption, and you'll lose weight. Combine that with exercise, and you'll lose more weight. In this chapter, I'll show you how my nutritional modification program can work for you regardless of how many pounds you want to shed.

While my philosophy is simple, it does require you to face some hard facts about your current dietary practices. You will be asked to count calories and fat grams in the beginning. By figuring the number of calories you need daily to maintain your current weight, you can estimate how many calories you should trim to lose pounds and how long you should exercise to burn a specific number of calories. This chapter will help you set realistic short- and long-term nutritional modification goals.

Then comes the easy part: putting your plan into action. The second half of this chapter contains a list of powerful, easy-to-use tips on how to eat smarter. After numerous false starts and failures, I realized that I could lower my calorie intake without feeling deprived and without diminishing my enjoyment of food, and I'll show you how to do that, too.

Step One

The first step is to calculate your break-even point: the number of calories your body needs each day to maintain its current weight. Body size, genetics, muscle-to-fat ratio, and metabolism (how fast the body burns calories) vary widely from person to person. It is difficult, therefore, to make a statement about calorie intake that will be accurate for everyone. But here is a formula I use as a general guideline:

$$\text{Weight} \times 15 = \text{Break-Even Point}$$

This means the human body needs about fifteen calories per pound per day to maintain its current weight. Adjustments should be made for age; you need one calorie less per pound per day during each ten-year period over age thirty. Here are some examples:

If you weigh 140 pounds and you're under age 30:

140 lbs. × 15 cals. = 2,100 cals./day

If you weigh 140 and you're 30 to 39:

140 × 14 = 1,960 cals./day

If you weigh 140 and you're 40 to 49:

140 × 13 = 1,820 cals./day

If you weigh 140 and you're 50 to 59:

140 × 12 = 1,680 cals./day

If you weigh 170 and you're 30 to 39:

170 × 14 = 2,380 cals./day

If you weigh 170 and you're 40 to 49:

170 × 13 = 2,210 cals./day

Step Two

Once you've calculated your break-even point, determine how many calories and fat grams you are consuming on a typical day. There is only one surefire way to do this: count calories. Buy a small notepad, or make photocopies of the calorie-counting chart (Chart 4.1) that appears in this chapter. Write down every food you consume and how many calories and fat grams it contains. Fill in your calorie log for a minimum of three days if you tend to eat the same foods every day, seven days if your cuisine is more eclectic. To obtain the most reliable results possible, don't alter your normal diet during these initial recording days. And don't bother recording on special occasions, such as weddings or Thanksgiving, when overeating is customary.

After your counting period is over, add each day's total to come up with a grand total, and divide it by the number of days you counted calories. Do the same for fat grams. These averages will give you a good idea of what you are putting into your body.

More important than knowing your average calorie consumption is knowing what percentage of your total calories comes from fat. Each gram of fat, regardless of its source, provides nine calories (compared to four calories per gram of carbohydrate). By multiplying your daily intake of fat grams by nine, you will know how many fat calories you consumed. Divide that number by your total calories to find out what percentage is fat.

Let's say, for instance, you take in 2,000 calories, including 50 grams of fat, during an average day. That's 450 fat calories, or about 22.5 percent of total calories. Not bad. If, however, your daily intake is 2,000 calories but you ingest 85 grams of fat, that's 765 fat calories or 38 percent, which is too high. As you become more conscious of the pitfalls in your current diet, you will be inspired to eat more healthfully.

I am the first to admit that calorie counting is a chore. But it is less of a chore than it used to be, thanks to the U.S. Food and Drug Administration. Several years ago, the FDA began requiring all packaged foods to include labels that clearly and uniformly summarize nutritional data. These data include the number of calories per serving, the number of fat grams, and what percentage of total calories those fat grams represent. Saturated fat grams also appear on labels, but I don't overly concern myself

---

Tip No. 18: Forgive Occasional Setbacks

●

If you fall off the wagon and skip one or more scheduled exercise sessions, don't assume your case is hopeless. Turn your guilt, anger, or disappointment into positive energy, and make a pact with yourself to get back into your fitness program as soon as possible.

Chart 4.1

●

CALORIE LOG

Day No. _____   **Date** _____

Food	Fat Grams	Total Calories

Breakfast:

_____	_____	_____
_____	_____	_____
_____	_____	_____

Lunch:

_____	_____	_____
_____	_____	_____
_____	_____	_____
_____	_____	_____
_____	_____	_____

Snacks:

_____	_____	_____
_____	_____	_____

Dinner:

_____	_____	_____
_____	_____	_____
_____	_____	_____
_____	_____	_____
_____	_____	_____
_____	_____	_____

Daily Totals: _____   _____

with the significance of different forms of fat. To me, fat is fat. I make a concerted effort to limit my intake of fat in all its forms.

When referring to food labels, please notice serving sizes. They may be smaller than you realize. Most restaurants, meanwhile, serve portions much larger than you need to fill you up. Like food manufacturers, restaurants and fast-food outlets are starting to make nutritional data available to customers. Eateries that offer lighter fare typically provide this information on the menu. If you don't find it, ask your server whether a calorie breakdown of menu items is available.

Chart 4.2 offers a list of selected popular foods and their calorie and fat contents. More comprehensive calorie-counting books are available at libraries, bookstores, and grocery-store checkout counters. One of the most comprehensive sources is *Bowes and Church's Food Values of Portions*

Chart 4.2

●

CALORIE/FAT GRAM CONTENT OF SELECTED FOODS

Food	Calories	Fat Grams
Coca-Cola (12 oz.)	144	0
Diet Coke (12 oz.)	1	0
Coffee (6 oz.)	4	0
Tea (6 oz.)	2	0
Orange juice (8 oz.)	104	0.4
Cranberry juice cocktail (6 oz.)	108	0.1
Country Time Lemonade (8 oz.)	82	0
Country Time Lemonade (sugar-free, 8 oz.)	5	0
Baby Ruth (2 oz. bar)	260	12.0
Butterfinger (2 oz. bar)	260	12.0
Cream of Wheat (¾ C)	100	0.4
Instant oatmeal (1 pkt.)	104	1.7
Cheerios (1 ¼ C)	111	1.8

(Continued on following page)

Food	Calories	Fat Grams
Golden Grahams (¾ C)	109	1.1
Grape-Nut Flakes	104	0.8
Puffed Wheat (1 C)	52	0.2
American cheese (1 oz.)	106	8.9
Cheddar cheese (1 oz.)	114	9.4
Philadelphia Cream Cheese (1 oz.)	98	9.5
Philadelphia Light Cream Cheese (1 oz.)	62	4.7
Mozzarella (1 oz.)	80	6.1
Part-skim mozzarella (1 oz.)	72	4.5
Half-and-Half Cream (1 T)	20	1.7
Boiled egg (1 large)	79	5.6
Scrambled egg w/milk, fat (butter or margarine)(1 large)	95	7.1
Egg Beaters (¼ C)	25	0
Kraft Macaroni & Cheese Delux Dinner (¾ C)	255	7.5
Spaghetti w/tomato sauce (1 C)	260	8.8
Spaghetti w/meatballs and tomato sauce (1 C)	332	11.7
Fish sandwich (fast food)	469	26.7
Hamburger (fast food)	245	11.1
Roast beef sandwich (fast food)	347	13.4
Mazola corn oil (1 T)	125	14.0
Mazola vegetable oil spray (2.5-sec. spray)	6	0.7
Van de Kamp's Light & Crispy Fish Sticks (4)	270	20.0
Baked flounder (3.5 oz.)	202	8.2
Breaded and fried shrimp (11 large)	206	10.4
Steamed shrimp (15 ½ large)	84	0.9
Apple (w/skin)	81	0.5

Food	Calories	Fat Grams
Banana	105	0.6
Fruit cocktail in heavy syrup (½ C)	93	0.1
Seedless raisins (⅔ C)	300	0.5
Bagel (plain)	163	1.4
Pita pocket	106	0.6
Whole wheat bread (1 slice)	61	1.1
English muffin (1 plain)	135	1.1
Homemade pancake (1 plain)	62	1.9
Boiled asparagus (6 spears)	22	0.3
Avocado (1 med.)	306	30.0
Boiled broccoli (½ c.)	23	0.2
Raw red cabbage (½ c. shredded)	10	0.1
Carrot (1 med.)	31	0.1
Raw cauliflower (½ c.)	12	0.1
Baked potato (w/skin)	220	0.2
Homemade potato salad (½ C)	179	10.3
French fries from restaurant (10 pieces)	158	8.3
Potato chips (1 oz.)	148	10.1
Pretzels (1 oz.)	111	1.0
Homemade brownie w/nuts (3" × 1" × ⅞")	97	6.3
Cheesecake (1 piece)	257	16.3
Homemade angel food cake	161	0.1
Chocolate chip cookie (2)	99	4.4
Fig Newton (2)	100	2.0
Ladyfingers (2)	79	1.7
Dole Strawberry Juice Bar (1)	70	0
Chocolate-coated Häagen-Dazs bar (1)	360	25.0

"Food Values of Portions Commonly Used" copyright © 1985, 1980 by Helen Nichols Church, B.S., and Jean A. T. Pennington, Ph.D., R.D. Reprinted with permission of HarperCollins Publishers, Inc.

Commonly Used, by Helen Nichols Church, B.S., and Jean A. T. Pennington, Ph.D., R.D. (HarperCollins). You can also find nutritional information (and meal ideas) in the plethora of low-fat cookbooks that line shelf after shelf in bookstores and libraries.

As you fill in your calorie diary, don't forget to include beverages and condiments. An eight-ounce glass of orange juice, while virtually fat free, has 112 calories. A glass of cola has 151 calories. Coffee may be calorie-free, but the cream and sugar you add to it are not. One tablespoon of butter will add 108 fat calories to your meal. A serving of water-packed tuna fish can be as low as 70 calories, but tuna salad made with mayonnaise contains more than 350 calories per serving.

Your calorie log is more than a document of your daily caloric intake; it can also be a motivational tool. Keeping the log will heighten your awareness of how many calories your favorite foods contain and which have the most fat grams. The log will help you think twice next time you reach for an ice-cream sandwich, and it should inspire you to scrutinize food labels in the grocery store.

Step Three

Once you know your break-even point, it is time to set some short- and long-term nutritional modification goals. If you are like the average American, the number of fat calories you take in probably exceeds 30 percent of total calories. If that is your case, make fat reduction a priority. I'm not saying that you should try to eliminate all fat from your diet. Going completely fat-free is extremely difficult and dangerous, since the body relies on small amounts of dietary fat to function normally. If your fat intake represents 40 percent of total calories, a worthy long-term goal would be to cut that in half—but not all at once. It is much easier to reduce fat gradually, by three or four grams a week, until you've met your long-term goal of 20 percent. So you don't have to stop eating ice cream; just don't eat the whole pint, or don't put as much chocolate sauce on it.

If you eat a steak at dinner, don't eat the whole thing—and have a piece of fruit for dessert. You'll feel better for it.

If you are consuming more calories than your break-even point requires, cutting your total calorie intake is a long-term goal worth shooting for. Here is where things get a little tricky, though. Simply cutting calories in the absence of regular exercise will not necessarily lead to weight loss. In fact, if you cut too many calories from your diet, you may have more difficulty shedding unwanted pounds. The reason lies in our genes. Human genetics have changed very little since our species was hunting and gathering food tens of thousands of years ago. Hunter-gatherers whose metabolism slowed down during times of famine survived because they didn't deplete their energy (fat) reserves before food became available again. That automatic survival mechanism was passed on genetically through the ages until it reached us. When we eat much less than we are accustomed to eating, physiologically our body thinks it is starving, so it slows down its metabolism to conserve energy. The net result is that the body burns less fat. Restricting your food intake also tends to intensify hunger, which can lead to eating binges.

There are a couple of ways to counteract this dilemma. One is to maintain your current calorie intake but replace some fat calories with carbohydrate calories. In other words, if you crave a sweet, have an apple or two, or even some jelly beans, instead of a chocolate bar. The body uses carbohydrate calories more efficiently than fat calories.

A second—and far superior—way to shift your metabolism into higher gear is to exercise. The importance of upping your physical activity a few weeks before you start cutting calories cannot be overempha-

---

Tip No. 20: Reward Yourself

You began your fitness program and stuck to it for two whole weeks. It's time to reward yourself—not with an ice cream soda but with a pair of athletic shoes, a new sweat suit, a CD you can play during your workout, or a new low-fat cookbook. Of course, it is unrealistic (and costly) to buy yourself a present after every exercise session, but rewarding yourself with a pat on your back and positive self-talk, such as "I did it!" and "Way to go!" is highly motivational. That is what I do for my clients. And I don't save all the accolades for the end of the session. Simply doing a particular exercise correctly or increasing your repetitions is a reason to slather yourself with praise.

sized. Not only do you burn calories during exercise but you also increase your muscle mass. The rear-end exercises, especially ones that include weights, will build that muscle. The higher your muscle-to-fat ratio, the more calories you will burn overall, even at rest.

Another way to build up muscle mass is to add more protein to your diet. Examples of high-protein, low-fat foods include egg whites, legumes, red meat and poultry, skim milk, water-packed tuna, and nonfat cottage cheese. Removing the skin from chicken and turkey and choosing the leanest cuts of red meat are easy ways to cut out fat.

While reducing fat and calories is important, don't cut out nutrition at the same time. Be careful to maintain a well-balanced diet. Eat a variety of foods every day, placing an emphasis on whole grains, fresh fruit, and vegetables. You should also drink eight glasses of water a day to help curb your appetite and prevent dehydration, especially in the summer.

ASSESSING VITAMINS, SUPPLEMENTS, AND POWDER DRINKS

As you eliminate or reduce certain foods from your diet, it is easy to sacrifice unwittingly some of the vitamins and minerals you need for good health. To make sure this doesn't happen, I take a multivitamin each day and recommend that you do the same.

I don't, however, take nutritional supplements, such as primrose oil, lecithin, ginseng, garlic oil, selenium, or chromium picolinate. Nutritional supplements are a multibillion-dollar-a-year industry. Unfortunately, the industry's success stems more from compelling advertising than from good science. The industry claims that supplements can build muscle, burn fat, or cure or prevent all sorts of medical problems, but in most cases, there is no conclusive scientific proof to support these claims. So unless your doctor orders you to take them, I think nutritional supplements are a waste of money.

The same goes for powdered drink mixes such as the egg-white protein powder sold primarily in health-food stores. These drinks may be high in protein, but most are also loaded with sugar and calories. Only very thin people who have difficulty gaining weight might benefit from these drinks.

Further, I join the chorus of medical and fitness professionals who oppose steroids and growth hormones as a means of building bigger, more vascular muscles. Steroid use not only carries significant health risks but also ignores the fitness trend of the nineties, which is not about being big. It's about looking athletic and natural and developing a body that looks sculpted, with a flat stomach and a nice rear end, but not one bristling with muscles and veins.

WHEN TO EAT?

Many of my clients ask me whether it is better to eat before or after exercising, and I can only tell them that I can run three miles after eating a major meal. Most people will become nauseous doing that, unless they are in excellent condition. You will probably feel better exercising on an empty stomach, thirty minutes to an hour after eating. If you are hungry before your scheduled workout, eat a complex carbohydrate such as a banana or other fruit, which is easily digestible and can provide the burst of energy you need. Do not eat a green salad prior to exercising because greens take a longer time to digest.

If you feel exhausted after exercising, complex carbohydrates, such as fruit, rice, pasta, baked potatoes, or vegetables, will pick your energy level back up. I also like to eat tuna fish with vinegar, sweet pickles, and no mayo, which is easily digestible and low in fat. If I am hungry after that, I will eat a frozen fruit bar, which has only seventy calories. If I am still hungry, I will eat another frozen fruit bar.

The idea is not to leave the table hungry but to satisfy your appetite with healthful foods. That was one of my long-term goals, along with not letting my daily fat intake exceed 20 percent of total calories or my total daily caloric intake top 1,500. After reaching those goals and combining them with a minimum of thirty minutes of exercise every day, I shed forty-eight pounds over six months. Since then, these goals have become part of me, just as your goals will become part of you.

Once you have set your goals, it is time to change your eating habits.

NUTRITIONAL MODIFICATION MADE SIMPLE

What follows are twenty-seven tips to help you reduce fat and calories in your diet. Not all suggestions will work for everyone, but chances are a few will work for you—and they may be all you need. Try one suggestion at a time. Continue the practices that feel most natural for you, and drop any that don't. Especially if you are used to a high-calorie, high-fat diet or you are more than thirty pounds overweight, I strongly advise against making radical changes in the beginning. You will have a better chance of long-term success if you ease into your nutritional modification plan. If you suddenly cut your calorie intake by 25 percent, you risk slowing down your metabolism and feeling so deprived that you won't be able to stick to your new dietary protocol.

I hope that you have already incorporated an exercise regimen into your lifestyle. If exercise is new for you, refrain from modifying your diet until exercising begins to feel natural. This waiting period is not wasted. If you maintain your current caloric intake but exercise at least three times a week, you will lose weight, although more slowly. Your weight loss will accelerate as soon as you combine exercise with calorie- and fat-cutting measures.

Here is my prescription for healthy eating:

1: CUT IT IN HALF. One of the least objectionable ways to reduce your fat intake is to make a policy of using half as much fat as you normally would use. Use a half pat of butter instead of a whole pat on your toast. Put two tablespoons of oil into your pasta sauce instead of four (each tablespoon contains at least 120 fat calories). Spread a thin coat of cream cheese on your bagel instead of a thick coat. Drink one glass of wine at dinner instead of two. Leave half of your dessert on the plate.

2: REPLACE FAT. As you learned from counting calories, fat grams add up very quickly. So any time you can replace a fat-filled food with a nonfat version, do it. Use skim milk and other fat-free dairy products. Try a dollop of fat-free yogurt or no-fat sour cream instead of butter on your baked potato. (Sweet potatoes are so creamy that they don't need butter at all.) Use fat-free yogurt in lieu of oil when making pancakes. Replace the cream cheese on your bagel with all-fruit jam.

3: MAKE A FAT RULE OF THUMB. Read food labels before buying anything. Reject items that derive more than 20 percent of calories from fat.

4: DON'T TEMPT YOURSELF. Rid your kitchen of ice cream, potato chips, and other fattening snacks. It is much easier to practice discipline in the grocery store than it is at home.

5: FORGIVE YOURSELF. Nobody's perfect. If you eat a cookie or fettuccine Alfredo, that doesn't mean you should throw your nutritional modification plan out the window. Forgive yourself and make a promise to get back to your diet beginning with your next meal.

6: TREAT YOURSELF TO A SWEET. Just because you are cutting back fat and calories does not mean you can't have dessert. Sorbet, fat-free ice cream, fat-free frozen yogurt, and frozen fruit bars are satisfying meal-enders. But remember that they may still be high in calories, so don't go overboard.

7: WAIT OUT THE CRAVING. When you have got to have chocolate, busy yourself with some project. Within thirty minutes or so, most junk-food cravings subside.

8: EAT SMALLER PORTIONS. Half a bowl of pasta can be just as satiating as a full bowl, especially after you've grown accustomed to eating less. Cut back your portions gradually, and stop eating as soon as you feel full. (When it comes to raw fruit and vegetables, however, eat as much as you like.) If you must have an Oreo, eat just one, and savor every morsel.

9: DON'T CLEAN YOUR PLATE. This runs contrary to what our mothers told us. Perhaps if we hadn't been compelled to finish every crumb when we were children, we wouldn't have such a hard time curbing our eating habits as adults. If you are worried about wasting food, save the leftovers for tomorrow's lunch.

10: PUT DOWN YOUR FORK. After each bite, put down your fork or spoon and give yourself a chance to chew and swallow before going for the next bite. This is an easy way to slow down the pace of your eating and give your digestive system a chance to tell your brain when your stomach is full.

11: DON'T GROCERY SHOP WHEN YOU ARE HUNGRY. You will be more tempted to buy fattening foods if your stomach is growling.

12: WHEN YOU ARE HUNGRY BETWEEN MEALS, RUN. Or swim, or walk, or jog in place, or ride your stationary bike, or do some rear-end exercises. Physical activity often curbs the appetite. If you are still hungry after exercising, eat with the satisfaction of knowing that whatever you consume will be burned off more quickly.

13: DON'T GET FOOLED. A fat-free food can still contribute a significant number of calories, so read food labels carefully.

14: WHEN YOU CRAVE SOMETHING FATTENING, LOOK IN THE MIRROR. Better yet, take off your shirt and look in the mirror. Ask yourself, "Is it worth it?"

15: KEEP HEALTHY SNACKS ON HAND. Every Sunday night, I wash a bag of baby carrots, cut up pieces of celery, and place these vegetables front and center in my refrigerator. I also put sliced strawberries in a bowl and sprinkle them with sugar. This way, when I feel like snacking during the week, I have fat-free munchies at my fingertips. Fat-free pretzels, apples and other fruit, air-popped popcorn (without butter, of course), fat-free caramel popped corn, fat-free oatmeal cookies, fat-free Fig Newtons, rice cakes, applesauce, gum, and mints are other low-calorie ways I quench my cravings. When I must have candy, I'll eat some Good & Plenty or jelly beans, both of which are fat-free.

16: AVOID UNCONSCIOUS EATING. Do you like to munch chips while chatting on the telephone, watching television, or driving? I call these habits "unconscious eating." If you are diligent about keeping your calorie log, you will become more conscious of these fattening habits.

17: EAT ONLY AT THE TABLE. Unconscious eating is easier to avoid if you make a rule to eat only at the table. This will also help you keep your calorie log. It's too easy to forget how much bread you put in your mouth while cooking dinner.

18: CUT BACK ON RED MEAT, OR SKIP IT. Ounce for ounce, most red meats have more fat and calories than poultry and fish. If you must eat red meat, choose the leanest cuts you can find and remove all visible fat before cooking. Grilled turkey burgers with mustard, tomato, and onion can be indistinguishable from hamburgers.

19: MAKE BREAKFAST FAT-FREE. Breakfast is the easiest meal when it comes to fat reduction. Most cold and hot cereals have no fat or just a trace. Pancakes can be made without oil or egg yolks and taste great when served with fruit in lieu of syrup and butter. Skip the butter on your oatmeal and mix in some skim milk and brown sugar instead. If you use whitener in your coffee or tea, try one of the new fat-free versions.

20: AVOID FRIED FOODS. If you do nothing else to curb your caloric intake, you can cut large amounts of fat and calories by avoiding fried foods, especially ones that are deep-fried—completely immersed in hot oil—such as french fries. Restaurants and fast-food outlets may try to hide the fact that a food is fried by calling it "breaded." Most restaurant chefs are happy to broil your fish or chicken on request.

21: NIBBLE. Research has shown that having a series of small meals and low-fat snacks throughout the day instead of three big meals can lower the level of low-density lipoproteins (LDL), the "bad" artery-clogging cholesterol, in your blood. Nibbling also increases your metabolism. Do your nibbling at the kitchen table whenever possible.

22: DON'T LET YOURSELF GET HUNGRY. Drink plenty of water, and eat at least five portions of raw fruits or vegetables every day.

23: DRINK TO YOUR HEALTH. With all the calorie-free sodas and iced teas on the market, there is no reason to add empty beverage calories to a meal. If you don't like the taste of diet sodas, try something else. Water is a perfect accompaniment to any meal.

24: BE A PARTIAL VEGETARIAN. If you normally eat meat or poultry for lunch and dinner, make one of those meals vegetarian.

25: DON'T EAT TO COPE WITH EMOTIONAL DIFFICULTIES. If you turn to food when you are depressed, bored, or lonely, find a more productive way to fill the void, such as exercise, a hobby, or volunteer work.

26: DON'T ADD FAT. As you saw from reading food labels, most packaged foods are made with some fat. Don't make matters worse by adding butter, margarine, or oil to foods. If you can't fathom bread without butter, try a different kind of bread, such as crusty French or Italian bread or fresh rye from a bakery, all of which are delicious on their own.

27: DON'T JUST THINK IT, DO IT. Nothing in this chapter should be new to you. Intellectually, we all know how to eat healthfully. But for many of us there is a mental block between knowing what to do and acting on this knowledge. To break through the block, continually remind yourself that your low-fat diet is a priority. When you begin to act on an impulse to eat a cookie or a bowl of ice cream, take a moment to think about what you are about to do. Is it worth it? Remind yourself that there are better ways to extinguish a craving or curb an appetite. If you believe that your nutritional modification goals are achievable, they will be.

SAMPLE MENU

Here is an example of a well-balanced, low-fat menu for a week.

SUNDAY

BREAKFAST: Blueberry pancakes made with skim milk; syrup; juice; coffee or tea

LUNCH: Fruit salad with fat-free cottage cheese or fat-free yogurt; lentil or split-pea soup (without ham); iced tea, seltzer, or water

SNACK: Banana

DINNER: Broiled swordfish marinated in fat-free dressing; steamed carrots, corn, or peas; fat-free pudding; iced tea or diet soda

MONDAY

BREAKFAST: Fat-free whole-grain cereal with skim milk; two slices whole-wheat toast with all-fruit jam; small glass of orange juice; coffee or tea

LUNCH: Bowl of tomato soup; tuna fish sandwich (made with low-fat or fat-free mayonnaise); carrot sticks; water or skim milk

SNACK: Two pieces of fresh fruit

DINNER: Broiled, skinless chicken breast; rice, peas, bread (optional); iced tea or seltzer

TUESDAY

BREAKFAST: Oatmeal; orange juice; glass of skim milk; coffee or tea

LUNCH: Chicken salad (made with fat-free dressing or vinegar) in tomato half; celery sticks; fat-free crackers; diet soda

SNACK: Two pieces of fresh fruit

DINNER: Broiled flank steak; baked potato (with fat-free yogurt); string beans; water, iced tea, or diet soda

WEDNESDAY

BREAKFAST: Whole-grain cereal with sliced banana and skim milk; fat-free yogurt; juice; coffee or tea

LUNCH: Three-bean salad; three pieces of melba toast with fat-free cheese spread; apple or pear; skim milk

SNACK: Peach slices with fat-free cottage cheese or fat-free yogurt

DINNER: Vegetable lasagna made with fat-free cheeses; green salad with low-fat or fat-free dressing; slice of Italian bread; water, iced tea, or diet soda

THURSDAY

BREAKFAST: Fat-free, whole-grain muffin with all-fruit jam; cup of fat-free yogurt topped with wheat germ; banana; juice; coffee or tea

LUNCH: Sliced turkey sandwich with mustard and lettuce; fat-free pretzels; piece of fruit; water, iced tea, or diet soda

SNACK: Frozen fruit bar

DINNER: Tossed salad with fat-free dressing; broiled salmon steak; rice; roll; fat-free pudding; water, iced tea, or diet soda

FRIDAY

BREAKFAST: Pineapple juice; spinach omelet made with egg substitute; fruit; coffee or tea

LUNCH: Grilled vegetables with vinegar on baguette; carrot sticks; water or seltzer

SNACK: Air-popped popcorn or fat-free pretzels

DINNER: Pasta and mixed vegetables in fat-free marinara sauce; calorie-free beverage; fat-free frozen yogurt

SATURDAY

BREAKFAST: Toasted bagel with all-fruit jam; skim milk; juice; coffee or tea

LUNCH: Sliced fat-free turkey breast on roll with honey mustard and tomato; skim milk or water

SNACK: Fruit or fat-free oatmeal raisin cookie

DINNER: Steamed vegetables with garlic on pasta or rice; diet soda or iced tea; slice of angel food cake or any fat-free cake

5

TRAINING TECHNIQUE

To get the most out of the rear-end exercises in this book, you must use correct form, or body positioning. This means distributing your weight properly, challenging the targeted muscle group to the utmost, and minimizing your risk of injury. In the fitness industry, these concepts are known collectively as "training technique"—and this technique is the focus of this chapter. Other aspects of training technique, such as warming up, cooling down, breathing, and proper weight-lifting form, will also be covered. In addition, this chapter will define exercise lingo such as "reps," "sets," and "overtraining." I will discuss the difference between normal muscle soreness and injury, and I will offer some home remedies for both. Finally, I will steer you toward the exercises that will help you reach your personal fitness goals, offering some advice on home exercise equipment as we go.

As mentioned earlier, progress toward your long-term and short-term goals will be quicker and more dramatic if you set a minigoal of working a little bit harder or a little bit longer each exercise session. Challenging yourself also prevents complacency. This chapter will provide tips on making the most of your workouts.

Tip No. 22: Don't Put Yourself Down

●

Are you the type of person who calls yourself "dummy" or "idiot" when you've made a mistake or failed at something? Negative self-talk can foster failure and lower self-esteem. Whenever you find yourself saying something negative about exercise or about your body, try to transform it into a positive statement. For instance, if you tell yourself you will never be fit enough to graduate to Stage Two exercises, change that to "As soon as I've mastered Stage One, I will be ready for Stage Two." If during a workout you tell yourself, "I can't go on," change that to "I know I can do this." If you say, "I'll always be too fat, no matter how much I exercise," transform the statement to "It took a long time to put on this extra weight. If I stick with the program, it will come off."

DETERMINING YOUR FITNESS LEVEL

Before learning more about training technique, and certainly before attempting any of the strength-training exercises in this book, you need to determine your current fitness level. Some readers will know instinctively what kind of shape they are in. If you are unsure, the following quiz should point you in the right direction. If you are still in doubt after taking the quiz, start with the least difficult training exercises. If these seem too easy or you experience absolutely no muscle soreness the day after your initial workout session, you probably need to increase the intensity of your workout or bump yourself up to the next stage.

If, on the other hand, you think your level is intermediate or advanced but you have difficulty executing the first Stage Two or Three exercises, then start with Stage One. If you cannot do any Stage One exercises, focus first on cardiovascular training and nutritional modification. In a couple of weeks, try some Stage One exercises again.

Do not feel embarrassed about being a beginner, and do not get discouraged. Instead, feel great about yourself for getting started; all you have to do now is stay with the program. You are not in competition with some faceless fellow reader who can run hurdles and complete twenty-five repetitions of every Stage Three exercise. If you are a beginner, you are in the majority, and that is why I have directed the bulk of this book toward you. If you follow my diet and exercise program diligently, I guarantee that you will move from a low fitness level to an intermediate level in six months or less. And there is a good chance that you will graduate to the advanced level less than a year from now.

FITNESS QUIZ

If you answer yes to one or more of the following questions, start with the Stage One exercises in Chapter Six:

Have you avoided regular workouts (at least twice a week) for the past six months or longer?

Are you 20 percent or more over your ideal weight?

Do you feel winded after walking up a flight of stairs?

Do you lead a mostly sedentary life?

Have you suffered a heart attack within the last three years?

Do you have lower back pain?

Do your bones ache?

Are you unable to bend over and touch your toes?

Are you a heavy smoker (a pack or more a day), or have you smoked for many years?

Have you made no serious attempts to lose weight through a combination of exercise and nutritional modification?

Are you unable to do one sit-up?

If you answer yes to one or more of the following questions, you are probably at an intermediate fitness level and can start with the Stage Two exercises in Chapter Seven.

Have you been working out regularly (at least twenty minutes three times a week) for the past three months?

Do you belong to a gym or fitness facility and use it regularly?

Are you able to jog at a moderate pace and at the same time carry on a conversation or sing out loud comfortably?

Can you swim ten laps in an Olympic-size pool without stopping?

Can you walk more than a mile without needing a rest?

Can you pedal a stationary bicycle nonstop for fifteen minutes?

Have you been playing at least one vigorous sport (such as singles tennis, racquetball, football, basketball, lacrosse, or soccer) at least once a week for the past six months?

If you answer yes to one or more of the following questions, you are probably at an advanced fitness level and can start with the Stage Three exercises in Chapter Eight.

Can you jog or run two miles without resting?

Do you consider yourself to be athletic?

Have you been working out regularly for more than a year?

Do you play a vigorous sport (such as singles tennis, racquetball, football, basketball, lacrosse, or soccer) three or more times a week?

Can you swim at least fifty laps in an Olympic-size pool without stopping?

ASPECTS OF TRAINING TECHNIQUE

When it comes to strength-training exercises like the ones in this book, proper form is absolutely essential. The best way to learn proper form is to watch someone else using it. Study the photographs in the following three chapters. If you can get your body in the same position my body is in when you begin and end each rear-end exercise, you will be using proper form. Use a mirror to check your form, or ask someone to look at the photos and coach you. Brief explanations accompanying each set of photographs reinforce where your hands, legs, feet, head, and other body parts should be in relation to one another or to the floor, and they tell you whether your back should be straight or curved.

It is vital to maintain proper form throughout each exercise's range of motion. Don't be surprised if proper form feels uncomfortable and awkward at first. My clients often have difficulty internalizing and executing proper form; like them, you will need time and practice before proper form feels like second nature.

Weight Distribution

If you are using proper form, then by definition, your weight will be properly distributed. This will help you keep your balance and train your muscles symmetrically.

If your weight is distributed correctly while doing the rear-end exercises, it will be easier for you to isolate your rear-end muscles. Proper weight distribution also reduces your risk of falling, pulling a muscle, putting unnecessary stress on a joint, or wasting energy training a muscle you are not focusing on. If I am doing a squat and my form is not good or if I am using too much weight, I can feel the pressure on my lower back and knees. As a beginner, you may feel some sensitivity in these areas even if your form is perfect. After a while, that sensitivity should ease off. If it doesn't, recheck your form.

Warming Up

The goal of warming up is to increase blood flow to your muscles. A few minutes of low-impact cardiovascular work or some gentle stretching will raise your body temperature a few degrees and increase blood flow to your muscles. This "priming the pump" makes muscles more flexible and prepares them for the challenges ahead. Warming up also reduces your risk of injury.

Regardless of whether you do cardiovascular activity before your exercises, I recommend these four gentle warm-up stretches. To avoid pulling a muscle, don't stretch aggressively, especially if your muscles are cold. If these stretches seem familiar, they are. In Chapter Three, I recommended the same stretches for cardiovascular workouts.

1: Stretch your arms out to your sides and do small clockwise circles for thirty to forty-five seconds. Then reach to the sky and out to your sides again and do counterclockwise circles for another thirty to forty-five seconds. This increases blood flow to your shoulder area.

2: Without turning your head, gently tilt your head from side to side three times and front and back three times. This increases flexibility in your neck area, a common injury site.

3: Bend over at the waist with your head down and try to touch your hands to the floor, your ankles, or your knees. Keeping your knees slightly bent, hang there for thirty to forty-five seconds. Don't bounce—bouncing can result in a pulled muscle if you are not warmed up. This bent-over stretch lengthens your lower back muscles and the muscles down the back of your legs. Round up out of the stretch very slowly, straightening up one vertebra at a time.

4: Placing your left hand on a wall for balance, bend your right knee, lifting your right foot up toward your rear. Grab your inner ankle with your right hand and pull your foot out behind you. Hold it for thirty seconds. Repeat with your other foot. This stretches your quadriceps (the front of your thighs).

Cooling Down

Repeating the same sequence of stretches after you complete your exercise session reduces your risk of cramping and soreness later. You will also find that your flexibility has increased markedly since your warm-up stretches.

Breathing

Developing a proper and consistent breathing pattern when doing strength-training exercise can take some practice. The key is to exhale during the exertion part of an exercise. If you are executing a squat, for example, inhale going down and exhale as you squeeze your rear-end muscles on the rise back up. Exhaling during the hardest part of an exercise cuts the chances of straining your diaphragm or something else inside. Never hold your breath during strength-training exercises. Your muscles need all the oxygen they can get. If you hold your breath, you can become dizzy or light-headed or may get a headache.

Weight Lifting

Several of the rear-end exercises require the use of free weights or weighted exercise machines. As a general rule, hold free weights fairly loosely in your hands. If you grip them too hard, you are wasting energy that can be better used training your rear-end and muscle groups surrounding muscle groups. Furthermore, by gripping too hard, your hands will fatigue before your rear end, and you won't be able to do as many repetitions as you could otherwise. When using weight-bearing exercise equipment, please follow the instructions in the exercise chapters.

Repetitions

The term *repetitions,* or "reps," stands for the number of times you perform a certain exercise. A single rep is the period from the beginning to the end of a particular exercise movement. For instance, a squat from the standing position down to the lowest position and back to the standing position equals one rep.

Sets

A *set* is the number of repetitions you can complete before resting. One set, for example, could be three, five, or ten reps. Generally, you want to do two or more sets of the same exercise, with rest periods in between, before moving on to another exercise. Another approach is to do one set each of five different exercises, then repeat the cycle. You don't necessarily have to complete the same number of reps in each set. Often you'll be able to do more reps the first set than in subsequent sets during any given workout.

Overtraining

If you develop muscle soreness that persists from workout to workout, you may be training a muscle group too hard; this is called *overtraining*. When you overtrain, you are breaking down muscle tissue instead of building it up. Russian weight lifters believe that the scar tissue formed as a result of overtraining ultimately makes the muscle stronger, but in the United States, overtraining is generally considered undesirable and potentially injurious. While it is difficult to overtrain the rear-end muscles since they are so massive, you can risk injuring something else, such as your knees, if you overtrain. Moreover, overtraining can lead to exercise burnout. So if your muscles are sore from exercise, wait until the soreness subsides before exercising that muscle group again.

Muscle Soreness

On the other hand, if you are not sore after training your rear end for the first time, you probably didn't work hard enough or long enough. Soreness, particularly when you begin a new exercise program, is absolutely normal. You are, in a sense, shocking your body, and that almost always results in some tenderness. In time, as your body becomes acclimated to exercise, the soreness will ease. Absence of normal soreness, however, can also mean that you are no longer making progress toward your fitness goals, and you should use this as a signal to try a new group of rear-end exercises, graduate to the next stage, increase your range of motion, increase the amount of weight you are lifting, squeeze your muscles a little harder, do the exercise a little slower, do more reps, or cut down your rest periods between sets.

Coping with Soreness

If your rear-end muscles are so achy that you are having trouble getting out of bed, sitting, and walking, you should refrain from the rear-end exercises for at least twenty-four hours. But that doesn't mean you can't do some cardiovascular work, such as swimming or walking, that doesn't overtax the gluteals.

Soaking in a hot bath or Jacuzzi or taking a hot shower after exercising can minimize soreness, as can gentle stretching and massage. Taking a couple of aspirin or ibuprofen (with food) can help. Rest is also therapeutic. Some nights I feel so sore that I cannot imagine working out again for at least two days. But if I go to bed an hour or two earlier than usual, I often wake up at 6:00 A.M. feeling totally recovered and ready to hit the gym.

Injury

If during exercise, you feel a sharp, shooting pain, stop. This probably means you pulled or strained a muscle or injured a joint. Pain on one side (unilateral) is another way to distinguish injury from normal muscle soreness, because normal soreness is almost always bilateral.

Coping with Injury

Never attempt to exercise through an injury. Instead, do some very gentle stretching of the injured muscle or joint, and focus the rest of your exercise session on a different muscle group. If you turn an ankle or incur some other kind of trauma during exercise, immediately ice and elevate the affected area to reduce swelling.

If you suffer an exercise injury, this probably means your form was off. To avoid future injuries, look at the pictures in the book again, check yourself out in a mirror, and fine-tune your form. Not warming up enough and overtraining muscles are other causes of injury.

Don't worry about falling off the wagon if you need to take a break from your strength-training exercises for a few days to let your injury heal. If you continue to do cardiovascular work and stick to your low-fat diet, you will continue to make progress.

HOW MANY REPS AND SETS SHOULD I DO?

The short answer is this: as many as you can. Repeat a given exercise until you feel your rear-end muscles burning, and then do two more. If you quit as soon as you feel the burn, it may take you twice as long to meet your goal. As your muscles grow stronger, it will take more reps to produce the burning sensation. A good rule of thumb is to increase your reps by one each time you work out.

   Use the log below to keep track of how many reps and sets you do. Don't forget to note if you are doing Stage One, Two, or Three exercises, since some of the exercises have the same names but different levels of

---

Chart 5.1

●

STRENGTH-TRAINING EXERCISE LOG

Week No._____

Dates_____to_____

Exercises	**Reps**	**Sets**
SUNDAY		
_____	_____	_____
_____	_____	_____
_____	_____	_____
_____	_____	_____
_____	_____	_____
_____	_____	_____
_____	_____	_____
_____	_____	_____
_____	_____	_____
_____	_____	_____

Exercises	Reps	Sets
MONDAY		
_____	_____	_____
_____	_____	_____
_____	_____	_____
_____	_____	_____
_____	_____	_____
_____	_____	_____
_____	_____	_____
_____	_____	_____
_____	_____	_____
_____	_____	_____
TUESDAY		
_____	_____	_____
_____	_____	_____
_____	_____	_____
_____	_____	_____
_____	_____	_____
_____	_____	_____
_____	_____	_____
_____	_____	_____
_____	_____	_____

Exercises	Reps	Sets
WEDNESDAY		
_____	____	____
_____	____	____
_____	____	____
_____	____	____
_____	____	____
_____	____	____
_____	____	____
_____	____	____
_____	____	____
_____	____	____
THURSDAY		
_____	____	____
_____	____	____
_____	____	____
_____	____	____
_____	____	____
_____	____	____
_____	____	____
_____	____	____
_____	____	____
_____	____	____

Exercises	Reps	Sets
FRIDAY		
_____	_____	_____
_____	_____	_____
_____	_____	_____
_____	_____	_____
_____	_____	_____
_____	_____	_____
_____	_____	_____
_____	_____	_____
_____	_____	_____
_____	_____	_____
SATURDAY		
_____	_____	_____
_____	_____	_____
_____	_____	_____
_____	_____	_____
_____	_____	_____
_____	_____	_____
_____	_____	_____
_____	_____	_____
_____	_____	_____
_____	_____	_____

intensity. You'll find that documenting your progress is a real confidence builder and a powerful motivator.

Counting Down

If you listen to the one-on-one trainers in my gym, you will hear more counting down of repetitions than counting up: they are using mental gravity. Just as it is easier to walk down a mountain than up a mountain, counting down is finite, while counting up can seem to take forever when you are working hard. Another trick is to count in groups. If you are doing twenty reps per set, for example, it will feel like fewer if you do two countdowns from ten.

Of course, you may count up if you prefer; it feels great looking down after you have reached the top of a mountain. The key here is to keep track of your reps so you can increase them next time.

Visualizing Your Muscles Contracting

Unlike cardiovascular training, which often begs for distractions such as TV or conversation to ward off boredom, effective strength-training work requires concentration and as few distractions as possible. This means putting on your answering machine and asking others to respect the precious time you have set aside for your workout. As you exercise, concentrate on keeping correct form and squeezing your rear-end muscles as hard as you can through the whole range of motion. Visualize your rear-end muscles working. Watch yourself in the mirror. Focus on your breathing. Count your reps out loud. Tell yourself you can do it. If you clear your mind of extraneous thoughts and really concentrate on what you are doing, exercise can become a form of meditation. When this happens, you are renewing your psyche even as you shape up your body. When your workout is over, you can't help but feel better about yourself and the world.

HOW LONG SHOULD I REST BETWEEN SETS?

The answer to this question depends on your fitness level and on how hard you are exercising. Beginners need to rest about forty-five seconds between sets. This should be enough time for the blood to carry away the lactic acid that builds up in the muscles you are exercising. As your fitness level improves, you should be able to decrease your rest period to thirty seconds in Stage Two and twenty seconds in Stage Three.

You'll need to increase your rest period slightly, however, if you are lifting heavier weights than you are used to or you are increasing your reps or the length of time you squeeze your muscles with each rep.

WHICH REAR-END EXERCISES ARE BEST FOR ME?

If you are female, you probably harbor most of your excess body fat on your rear end, hips, and thighs. If your rear end sags and you want to make it higher, select exercises that work the entire rear end directly and the lower back indirectly. Your choices include back leg lifts, the half squats (close and wide stance), the Smith squat, and the cable leg kick backs. If you want to slim down and tone up your inner thighs, do exercises that work the inner thighs directly. These include the Buttock Lift, Wide Stance (No. 2); Leg Lift to Side (No. 17); Knee In, Leg Up (No. 5); the Full Lunge (No. 12); and Straight Leg Lifts (No. 14).

Do at least three different rear-end exercises three times a week. To burn more calories, do as many reps as you can as fast as you can without sacrificing form. To increase the intensity of your workouts, simply do more reps or sets or add another exercise. Free weights, which are used in some Stage Two and Three exercises, should be light—three to five pounds. Don't worry about your rear-end muscles "bulking up" if you exercise hard. If you are female, your hard work will pay off with a firmer, stronger behind and a shapelier figure.

In addition to the rear-end exercises, you'll need to complete at least three fat-burning cardiovascular workouts a week. If you haven't engaged in aerobic exercise regularly for six months or longer, start with a ten-

---

Tip No. 23: Log Your Progress

●

Some people like seeing things in black and white to prove to themselves they are making progress. If you are one of those people, you may find it helpful to keep an exercise log. An exercise log helps you remember how much you did each workout session so you can increase the intensity the next time. At my gym, the personal trainers keep logs for all our clients. If clients get discouraged, they can look at their logs to remind themselves how far they have come.

minute workout. Increase the next week's workout session to ten and a half minutes, then eleven, and so on until you are able to exercise for forty-five minutes. As you get stronger, you'll also be able to increase your workout frequency to four times a week, then five.

Men tend to carry excess fat on their abdomen, not their rear end. If you are male and want to reduce the size of your gut and also tone your rear, focus first on cardiovascular work and calorie cutting.

If your rear end is too small, do fewer reps but use heavier weights or hold each squeeze an extra long time. Again, beginners should start slowly in Stage One with a goal of increasing the weight and length of time you hold each squeeze as you move on to Stage Two exercises and, later, Stage Three. The amount of muscle tone you develop depends on how much weight you use in your strength-training workouts, how many different rear exercises you do each session, and how hard you are able to squeeze your muscles. Remember, use as much weight as you can handle without sacrificing proper form. Any of the rear exercises that work all the gluteal muscles directly will help you develop a more muscular, rounded rear end.

At the beginning of each exercise chapter, you will find more recommendations on how to create your own routine based on my prescription.

MAKING EVERY EXERCISE SESSION COUNT

There are a variety of ways to increase the intensity of every workout:

- Add another exercise to your routine each week.
- Increase reps by one or two.
- Decrease the rest period between reps.
- Decrease the rest period between sets.
- Squeeze your rear muscles a little harder or a little longer.
- Juggle the rear-end exercises so you do a different group each day.
- If you have been doing Stage One exercises for two months, throw in a Stage Two exercise. If you've been in Stage Two, add one of the Stage Three exercises.
- Exercise two minutes longer.
- Use slightly heavier weights.

- Increase the number of days per week you exercise.

- For cardiovascular work such as jogging, add another thirty seconds per session or jog a little faster than you did the time before.

- Push yourself to your limit each time you work out.

- Use your mind-body connection to visualize your muscles squeezing tighter and getting stronger.

- Dress warmly when you work out. Wear sweats or at least drape a towel around your neck. The body has to work harder and burn more calories when its temperature is elevated.

HOW FREQUENTLY SHOULD I EXERCISE?

When some people launch into an exciting new exercise program, they expect immediate gratification, so they exercise to exhaustion seven days a week. This is a prescription for burnout. My advice is to pace yourself; don't feel compelled to train your rear-end muscles on a daily basis, even if the exercises you are doing are not intense. Strength training three times a week, if coupled with calorie cutting, will ultimately change the size and shape of your rear end. Devote two or three days to cardiovascular work, even if it is only walking in place in front of your television set. As you saw in Chapter Three, there are many unexpected sources of aerobic activity that you can exploit with relative ease.

HOW LONG SHOULD MY EXERCISE SESSION LAST?

In the case of cardiovascular training, you should exercise with your heart rate in its target zone for a minimum of twenty minutes per workout. Add to that about five minutes to warm up and another five minutes to cool down. The longer you can sustain your aerobic workout, the more fat you'll burn—from your rear end and the rest of your body. I like to run on a treadmill and can do so for a solid forty-five minutes. If you are not used to aerobic exercise, don't get down on yourself if you can run for only ten minutes at first. If you don't give up, it will get easier. And remember, you needn't exercise to exhaustion. Once your heart rate reaches its target zone, you should be able to carry on a conversation as you continue your workout.

The effectiveness of your strength-training workout depends on how hard you squeeze your muscles and how long you are able to sustain the squeeze as opposed to the overall length of your exercise session. If you're a beginner, hold the squeeze for at least three seconds per rep. Intermediate exercisers should try to hold the squeeze for at least five seconds. Advanced exercisers should shoot for a ten-second squeeze per rep.

If you are just starting out, do ten minutes' worth of Stage One exercises two or three times the first week. The next week, increase that to eleven minutes, then twelve, and so on. Eventually, you'll be strong enough to do strength-training exercises for twenty minutes three times a week.

ROTATION TRAINING

As mentioned in Chapter Two, the rear end's muscle group is comprised of three distinct yet interconnected muscles: the gluteus maximus, gluteus medius, and gluteus minimus. In order to make your buttocks tighter and more uplifted, you must regularly challenge all of the gluteal muscles, as well as the surrounding muscles of the thighs, lower back, and abdomen. The best way to do this without undue muscle fatigue and soreness is by rotation training. By rotating a variety of exercises in and out of

---

Tip No. 24: Throw Out Your Scale

When people set weight-loss goals for themselves, they often gauge their progress strictly by the scale. If the numbers don't go down enough after several months of hard work and discipline, some people ask themselves, "What's the use?" and quit.

First, no one but you (and perhaps your physician) needs to know how much you weigh. Second, muscle tissue is denser and heavier than fat tissue. That is why obese people float easily in swimming pools while people with muscular physiques sink like stones. If you are losing fat and gaining muscle as you follow my program, your weight could stay the same or even go up. The true tests are your mirror and wardrobe. Does your body look tighter? Are clothes that were once snug beginning to fit better? Have you dropped a dress size? If you stick with my program, I guarantee you'll be answering yes to all those questions.

each workout session, you'll hit all your target muscle groups from every possible angle.

To help you decide which exercises to do, look at the part of the exercise description that tells you which muscles are targeted directly and indirectly. Be sure to read through all the exercises in a particular chapter before selecting at least three that alternately focus on the entire rear and specific portions of the rear. Avoid doing more than three exercises in a row that directly hit the same muscle groups.

Depending on how much time you rest between sets (beginners generally take about forty-five seconds), the strength-training sessions should last fifteen to twenty minutes.

Here is an example of a Stage One workout schedule that includes three strength-training workouts and three cardiovascular workouts over the course of a week. It is designed for a beginner. Remember, repeat each exercise until you feel the burn, then do at least two more. Rest until the burn subsides and repeat.

Monday

No. 1: Buttock Lift, Close Stance (works entire rear directly; inner and outer thigh indirectly)

No. 2: Buttock Lift, Wide Stance (works lower and outer rear and inner thigh directly; abdominals and lower back indirectly)

No. 10: Step-up Lunge (works lower rear end directly; middle and upper rear and hamstrings indirectly)

Tuesday

Power-walk for thirty minutes

Wednesday

Day of rest

Thursday

No. 8: Back Leg Extensions (works entire rear and hamstrings directly; inner and outer thigh indirectly)

No. 15: Straight Leg Lifts, Toe Pointed (works lower rear, quadriceps, outer and inner thigh directly; middle and upper rear end and hamstrings indirectly)

No. 1: Buttock Lift, Close Stance (works entire rear directly; inner and outer thigh indirectly)

Friday

Power-walk or walk in place for thirty minutes

Saturday
No. 1:   Buttock Lift, Close Stance (works entire rear directly; inner and outer thigh indirectly)
No. 2:   Buttock Lift, Wide Stance (works lower and outer rear and inner thigh directly; abdominals and lower back indirectly)
No. 17:   Standing Leg Lift to Side (works entire rear and outer and inner thigh directly; hamstrings and quadriceps indirectly)

Sunday

Power-walk or walk in place for thirty minutes

Another option is to do your strength-training workout in the morning and your cardiovascular workout in the evening (or vice versa) three days a week.

HOME EXERCISE EQUIPMENT

If you intend to stick with your exercise program indefinitely (and I hope you do), but you don't want to join a fitness center, you may wish to consider investing in some home-exercise equipment. Exercise equipment can be expensive and may take up precious room in your house or apartment. But there are several important advantages to owning your own equipment: you can exercise whenever you want, the per-use cost goes down the more you use it, you can exercise in private, you can get other family members involved, and you don't have to pay an annual membership fee.

Strength-Training Equipment for the Home

Beginners need not worry about home exercise equipment until they reach the intermediate and advanced levels. Most of the Stage Two and Three rear-end exercises use free weights (a barbell and dumbbells), and several exercises require weight machines. Exercise machines allow you to work out with heavier weights safely.

Everyone at the intermediate or advanced fitness levels should have access to a set of "plate-loaded" dumbbells, which allow you to increase or decrease the amount of weight you are lifting. The plates are kept on with a metal "collar." You can buy plate-loaded dumbbells at most sporting goods stores for about five dollars a pound, and every fitness center should have them.

Modern home-exercise machines have become fairly streamlined. The best value is to buy a "multipurpose station," which can be reconfigured to work all the major muscle groups, including the rear end. I recommend the Soloflex, which retails for about $500. I also recommend multipurpose stations made by Universal or Cybex, which offer up to twenty-five different exercises. They range in price from about $2,500 to $10,000. A good machine is expensive, but this in turn gives you a financial motivation for improving your health. And in the long run, owning your own exercise machine can be less costly than joining a fitness center.

Cardiovascular Exercise Machines for the Home

Of course, the simplest and least expensive aerobic workout at home consists of power-walking or jogging in place or dancing on your living-room floor.

Nonetheless, millions of people at every fitness level have purchased a treadmill, stationary bicycle, stair-climbing machine, rowing machine, ski machine, or other piece of cardiovascular equipment. You can spend anywhere from $100 to $1,000 or more for one of these machines, and each year manufacturers introduce more choices. Generally, the more the machine costs, the better its quality. However, many of the bells and whistles—pulse monitors, digital odometers, speedometers, and calorie counters—do little but jack up the price. You can take your own pulse and use a watch to time your workouts. You don't need to know your "speed" or "distance" so long as your heart rate is in its target zone and you have broken a sweat. Built-in calorie counters are unreliable because people burn calories at different rates, depending on their metabolism and fitness level.

Before buying anything, visit several sporting goods stores and try out as many floor models as you can. Your goal is to find something you enjoy and feel comfortable with. Steer clear of items whose floor sample is beat up or broken. If the floor model can't stand up to the abuse it gets while on display, the machine probably won't serve you well at home.

When using your cardiovascular equipment at home, keep a water bottle close at hand so you don't have to stop and dismount every time you want a drink. Follow the machine's instructions carefully, especially on an automatic treadmill, which can be dangerous if you lose your footing.

Secondhand Exercise Equipment

You can save a few dollars by purchasing secondhand machines. Some retail chains specialize in "previously owned" exercise equipment. Another source is your local newspaper's classified advertising section. Make sure the machine is sturdy and that there are no missing nuts or bolts. Try out the machine, paying close attention to how smoothly the mechanism responds. In the case of strength-training equipment, be sure that all the original add-on weights are present. You don't want to force yourself to lift too much or too little weight because some pieces of equipment are missing.

A main advantage to home-exercise equipment is that it helps eliminate excuses for not working out. The machine also symbolizes your long-term commitment to exercise. Your willingness to make a financial investment in your health should motivate you to use the equipment as often as possible.

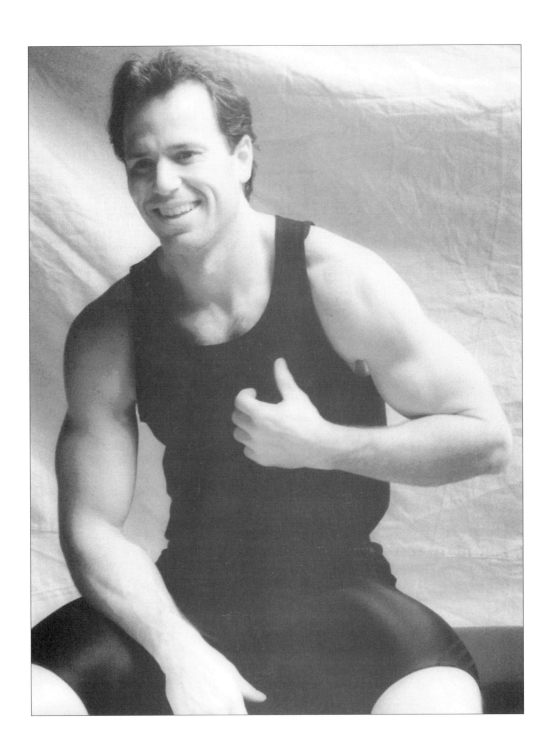

6

STAGE ONE: BEGINNER REAR-END EXERCISES

I enjoy training people of all fitness levels, but my favorite clients are the beginners. Why? Because I am able to teach them good form right off the bat without having to break their bad habits. If you have never tried strength-training exercises before and do not know where to begin, the rear end is a perfect starting point. The twenty-four Stage One exercises that follow are designed for people who have never trained this muscle group before or who otherwise consider themselves sedentary or out of shape.

In order to make the greatest impact on your rear end, you must use the same form I use in the "before" and "after" photographs that illustrate each exercise. Do each repetition slowly while visualizing your muscles squeezing. The object here is to isolate and strengthen your rear-end muscles, not necessarily to burn fat or give your heart a workout. Exhale during the exertion phase of each exercise. Practice talking yourself through each exercise, counting each rep, saying out loud such statements as "Come on, you can do it," and "Way to go!" Turn on some music, if that will help motivate you.

Most of the Stage One exercises are "manual exercises," which means they require no equipment. One of the exercises, the Step-up Lunge (No.

10), requires a six-inch step. You can use a small step stool or large telephone book. The exercises that require equipment are optional. Wherever you are when you do your strength-training exercises, be sure you always exercise on a mat or carpeted floor.

GETTING STARTED

Having read this far in the book, you are probably eager to get started. I admire your enthusiasm; it is a vital component of motivation. But please do not get carried away. Start these exercises gradually; don't go overboard the first couple of sessions.

The first step is to look at all the Stage One exercises and select three to five you would like try the first week. Write the exercises' names or number designations in your Exercise Log (Chart 5.1). The exercises are presented roughly in order from the least difficult to the most difficult. Make a short-term goal of mastering these three to five exercises during week one. Then do three to five different Stage One exercises each subsequent week until you have mastered them all. As proper form begins to feel more comfortable, you will be able to choreograph different exercise combinations each time you work out. This approach keeps your workouts fresh and interesting. Be sure to warm up before each workout with the gentle stretches described in Chapter Five.

If you have never trained your rear end before, do not force yourself to do more than one set per exercise in the beginning. Do your first exercise over and over until you feel a burning sensation in your rear end. The burn signals a buildup of lactic acid associated with muscle fatigue. Rest for about forty-five seconds or until the burn subsides. Then move to the next exercise and repeat the process. Some exercises, like the Quarter Plié (No. 7), work both sides of the rear end simultaneously. Others, like the Back Leg Extensions (No. 8), train one side of the muscle group at a time. For such exercises, complete as many repetitions as you can on one side before moving to the other. Do the same number of reps on each side so your muscles will be trained symmetrically. You will burn up to ten calories per minute if you do the rear-end exercises as quickly and intensely as you can.

After finishing each exercise, jot down in your Exercise Log the number of repetitions you did. Some beginners will be able to complete ten or more reps per exercise. But do not be discouraged if you can do only four or five reps at first. After all, you're doing more than you did last week. If you train for fifteen minutes a day for three days during week one and use proper form, I guarantee you will be able to increase your repetitions the second week. As you get stronger, you will also be able gradually to reduce your rest periods and increase the number of exercises you do. Every now and then, double-check your form and breathing pattern. Are you squeezing your rear end throughout the entire range of motion? Are you squeezing a little harder than you did during your last workout session?

Beginning with week two, start pushing yourself to do one or two reps beyond the burn. This way you will make progress gradually without putting undue stress on your body. You might be surprised at how fast your muscles respond. When you can complete twenty consecutive reps of a particular exercise, add a second set of five reps. Increase the number of reps in the second set by one each session until you reach twenty. Develop your third set the same way. When you can do three twenty-rep sets of eight Stage One exercises, you are ready to advance to Stage Two. Or you can ease into Stage Two by adding some intermediate exercises to your Stage One routine.

1

BUTTOCK LIFT, CLOSE STANCE

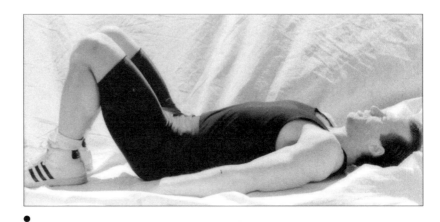

● **STARTING POSITION:**
Lie on your back with your knees bent, knees and feet together, hands down to side on floor, and back flat.

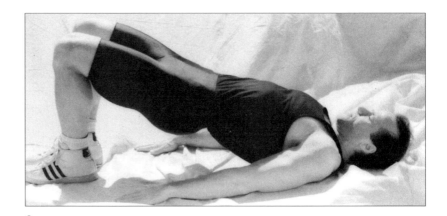

● **ACTION:**
Keeping rear end tight, lift rear end and upper back off floor as high as you can, squeezing rear-end muscles as hard as you can. Hold two seconds. Lower slowly to starting position.

● **MUSCLES WORKED DIRECTLY:**
Entire rear end (gluteus maximus, medius, and minimus)

● **MUSCLES WORKED INDIRECTLY:**
Inner and outer thigh (adductor, sartorius, tensor fasciae latae)

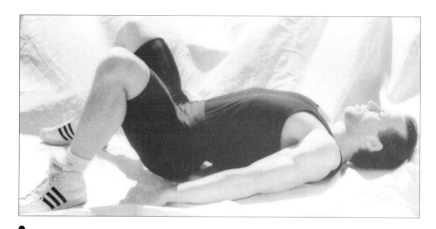

2

BUTTOCK
LIFT,
WIDE
STANCE

STARTING POSITION:
Lie on your back with your knees bent, knees and feet about shoulder width apart, back slightly arched, hands to side.

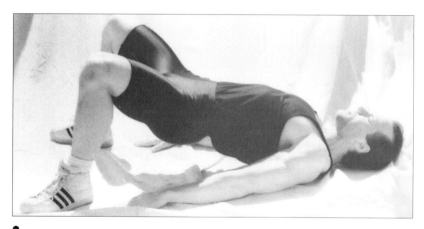

ACTION:
Squeezing the rear end as hard as you can, lift rear and lower back. Hold two seconds. Lower slowly to starting position.

● **MUSCLES WORKED DIRECTLY:**
Lower and outer rear end (gluteus maximus), inner thigh

● **MUSCLES WORKED INDIRECTLY:**
Abdominals (rectus abdominis and external obliques), lower back (latissimus dorsi), back of thigh (hamstrings)

3

HIP RELEASE AND STRETCH

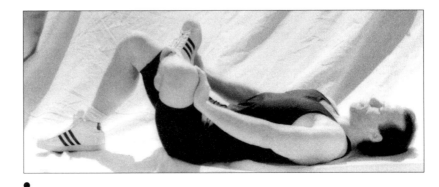

STARTING POSITION:
Lie on your back. Keeping back flat, cross left leg over right thigh and gently push left hand on left knee and stretch for ten seconds.

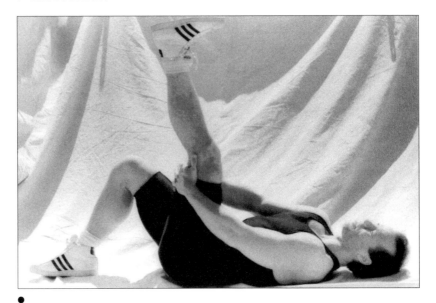

ACTION:
Squeezing rear end as hard as you can, straighten left leg, clasping both hands behind knee. Pull and stretch gently for ten seconds. Repeat with right leg.

● **MUSCLES WORKED DIRECTLY:**
Entire rear end

● **MUSCLES WORKED INDIRECTLY:**
Hamstrings

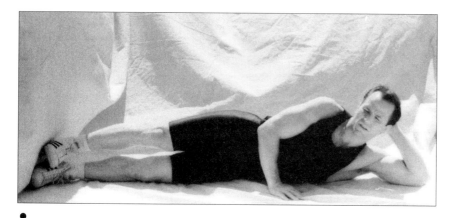

4

LEG LIFTS
TO SIDE

● **STARTING POSITION:**
Lie on your side, relax bottom leg and foot, flex toes of upper foot, support head with hand.

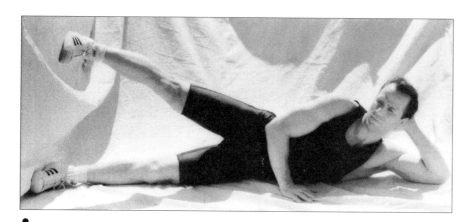

● **ACTION:**
Keeping leg and rear-end muscles tight, lift top leg as high as you can. Hold two seconds. Return to starting position.

● **MUSCLES WORKED DIRECTLY:**
Outer thigh, upper and lower rear end

● **MUSCLES WORKED INDIRECTLY:**
Inner thigh, abdominals

5

KNEE IN, LEG UP

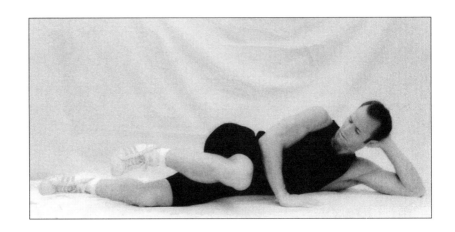

STARTING POSITION:
Lie on your side, back straight, resting head on hand. Bend knee of top leg and flex foot, keeping it parallel to the floor throughout exercise. Bottom leg may be slightly bent.

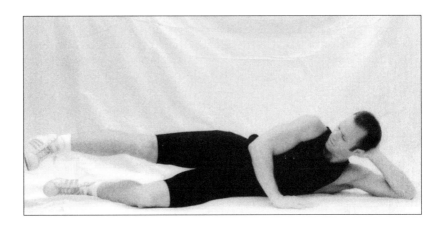

ACTION:
Straightening knee, raise top leg as high as you can. Hold two seconds. Return to starting position.

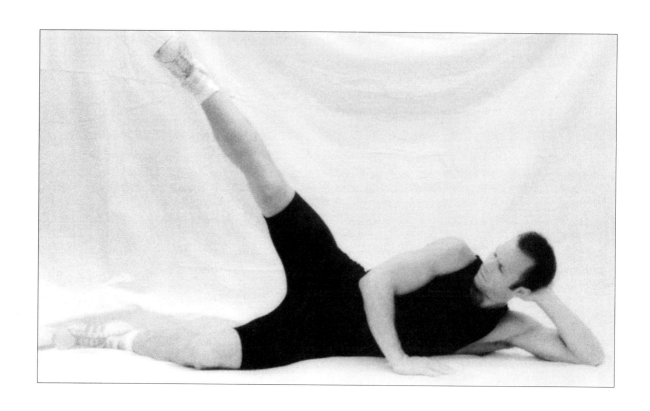

● **MUSCLES WORKED DIRECTLY:**
Lower rear end, outer thigh

● **MUSCLES WORKED INDIRECTLY:**
Inner thigh, hamstrings

6

BACK LEG LIFTS

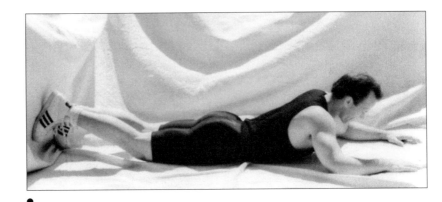

STARTING POSITION:
Lie on your stomach, hands out in front, head and feet slightly raised.

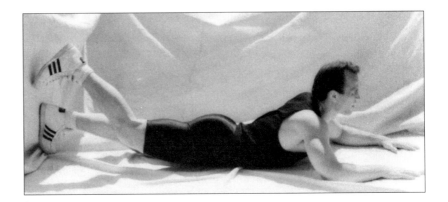

ACTION:
Keeping left leg slightly bent, lift it as high as you can. Hold two seconds, squeezing the rear end as hard as possible. Return to starting position.

● MUSCLES WORKED DIRECTLY:
Entire rear end

● MUSCLES WORKED INDIRECTLY:
Hamstrings, lower back

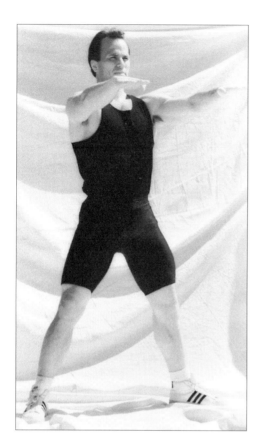

STARTING POSITION:
Stand with feet flat, toes pointed out, knees slightly bent, hands on hips or out in front for balance.

QUARTER PLIÉ, WIDE STANCE

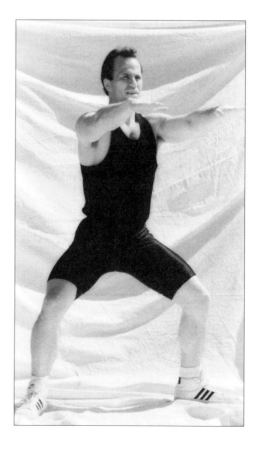

ACTION:
Keeping heels on floor, squat slightly, squeezing rear-end muscles. Hold two seconds. Return to standing position.

● **MUSCLES WORKED DIRECTLY:**
Entire rear end

● **MUSCLES WORKED INDIRECTLY:**
Hamstrings, inner and outer thigh

8

BACK LEG EXTENSIONS

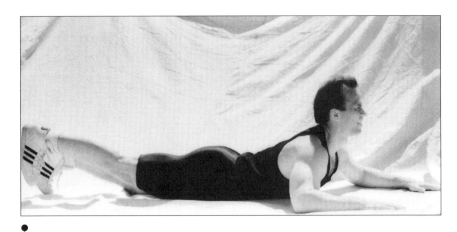

STARTING POSITION:
Lie on stomach, hands extended out front, head raised, left foot raised slightly.

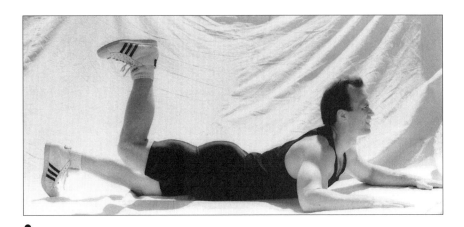

ACTION:
Squeezing rear end, bend left knee, keeping foot flexed. Hold two seconds. Lower leg to floor.

● **MUSCLES WORKED DIRECTLY:**
Entire rear end, hamstrings

● **MUSCLES WORKED INDIRECTLY:**
Inner and outer thigh

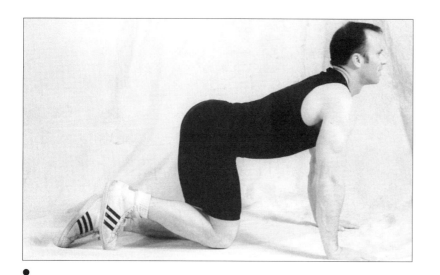

9

MULE KICKS

● **STARTING POSITION:**
On hands and knees, keep lower back flat, head up, elbows locked, feet and knees together.

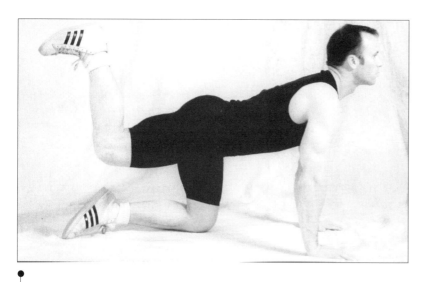

● **MUSCLES WORKED DIRECTLY:**
Entire rear end, hamstrings

● **MUSCLES WORKED INDIRECTLY:**
Inner and outer thigh

● **ACTION:**
With foot flexed and knee bent, lift left leg as high as you can, squeezing rear end. Hold two seconds. Return to starting position. Repeat on the other side.

10

STEP-UP LUNGE

(Six-inch step required)

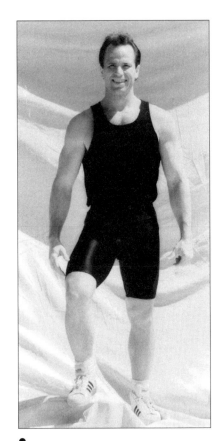

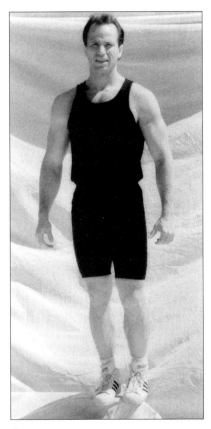

STARTING POSITION:
Stand with right foot on six-inch step, left foot on floor about one foot behind right foot, hands to your side or in front of you for balance.

ACTION:
Stepping up onto right foot, place left foot on step. Hold two seconds, squeezing rear-end muscles tightly. Bring right foot back to floor behind you, and repeat on the other side.

● **MUSCLES WORKED DIRECTLY:**
Lower rear end

● **MUSCLES WORKED INDIRECTLY:**
Middle and upper rear end, hamstrings

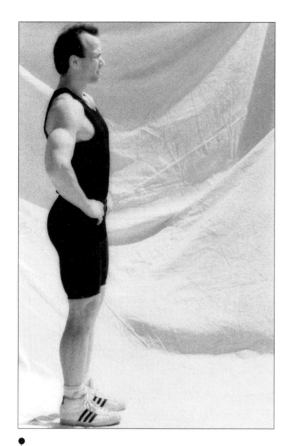

PARTIAL LUNGE, NO WEIGHT

STARTING POSITION:
Stand with legs together, toes pointing forward, knees slightly bent, hands on hips.

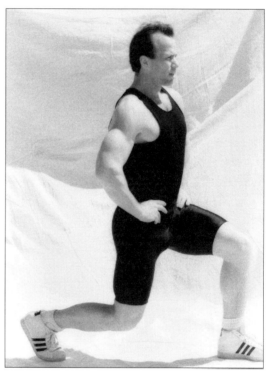

ACTION:
Keeping rear end tight, step forward with left leg. Keeping left foot flat on the floor at all times, bend back knee toward floor (but don't touch floor), putting your weight on toes of back foot. Return to starting position.

● **MUSCLES WORKED DIRECTLY:**
Entire rear end, hamstrings

● **MUSCLES WORKED INDIRECTLY:**
Inner and outer thigh

12

FULL LUNGE, NO WEIGHT

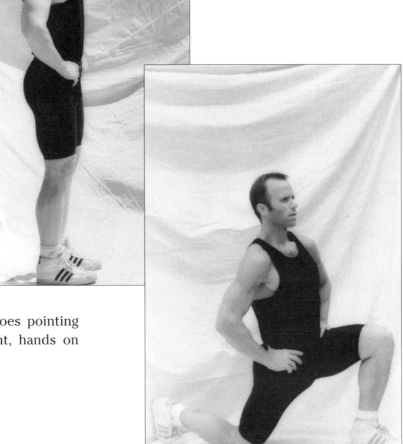

STARTING POSITION:
Stand with legs together, toes pointing forward, knees slightly bent, hands on hips.

ACTION:
Keeping rear end tight, step forward with left leg. Keeping left foot flat on the floor at all times, bend back knee to touch floor, put weight on toes of back foot. Return to starting position.

● **MUSCLES WORKED DIRECTLY:**
Lower rear end, outer thigh

● **MUSCLES WORKED INDIRECTLY:**
Inner thigh

Get Your Rear in Gear

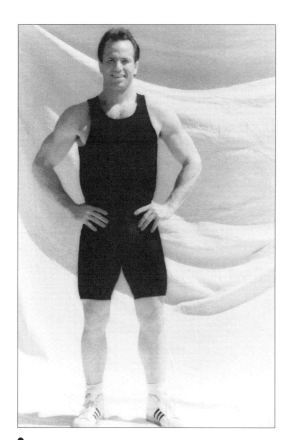

13

SIDE LUNGE

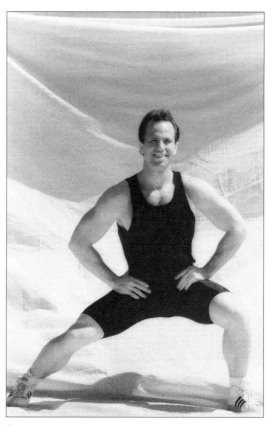

● STARTING POSITION:
Stand with knees slightly bent, feet slightly apart, hands on hips or to side for balance.

● MUSCLES WORKED DIRECTLY:
Entire rear end, hamstrings

● MUSCLES WORKED INDIRECTLY:
Inner and outer thigh

● ACTION:
With right leg, step straight out to side with toes pointed out slightly as you bend your left knee. Return to starting position.

14

STRAIGHT LEG LIFTS, FOOT FLEXED

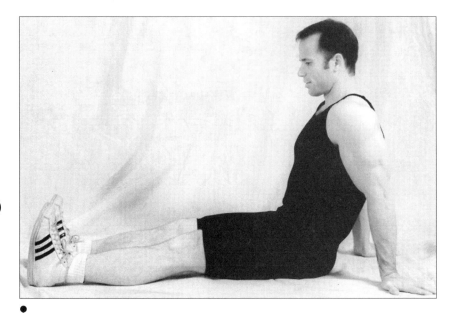

STARTING POSITION:
Sit on floor, hands flat on floor behind you, feet turned out with knees slightly bent, feet flexed.

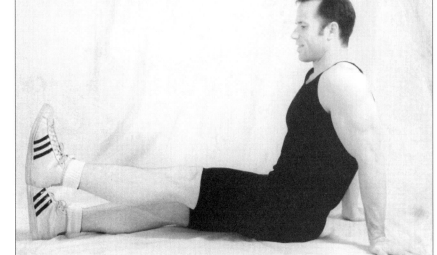

● **MUSCLES WORKED DIRECTLY:**
Lower rear end, hamstrings, outer and inner thigh

● **MUSCLES WORKED INDIRECTLY:**
Middle and upper rear end

ACTION:
Keeping knees slightly bent and foot flexed, raise left leg as high as you can. Hold two seconds. Return to starting position.

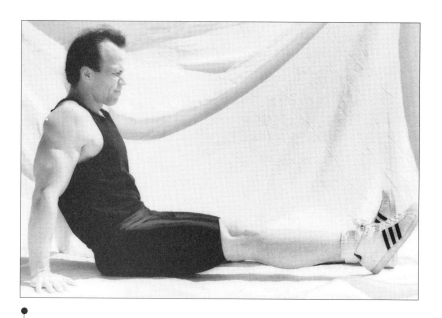

STRAIGHT LEG LIFTS, TOE POINTED

STARTING POSITION:
Sit on floor, hands flat on floor behind you, feet turned out with knees slightly bent, left toe pointed.

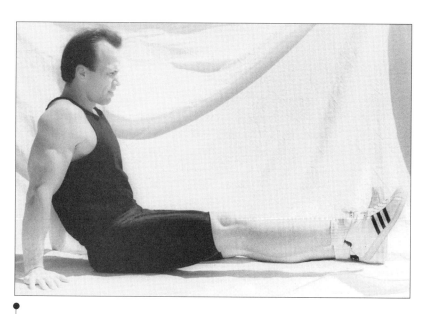

● **MUSCLES WORKED DIRECTLY:**
Lower rear end, front of thigh (quadriceps), outer and inner thigh

ACTION:
Keeping knees slightly bent and toe pointed, raise left leg as high as you can. Hold two seconds. Return to starting position.

● **MUSCLES WORKED INDIRECTLY:**
Middle and upper rear end, hamstrings

16

SIDE LEG LIFT TO FRONT

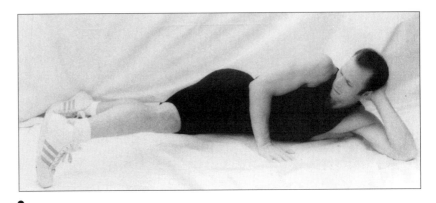

● **STARTING POSITION:**
Lie on side, supporting head with hand. Top leg is forward with toe on floor; bottom leg and foot are resting on floor.

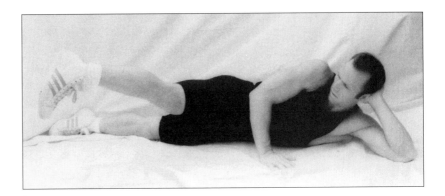

● **ACTION:**
Without changing angle of top foot, lift top leg nine to twelve inches off floor. Return to starting position, but do not allow toe to touch the floor between reps.

● **MUSCLES WORKED DIRECTLY:**
Upper rear end, hamstrings

● **MUSCLES WORKED INDIRECTLY:**
Lower and middle rear end, quadriceps

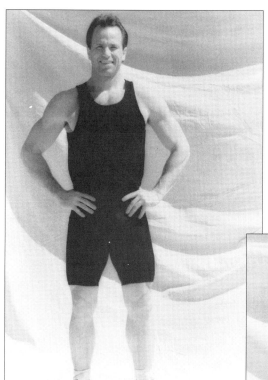

17

STANDING
LEG LIFT
TO SIDE

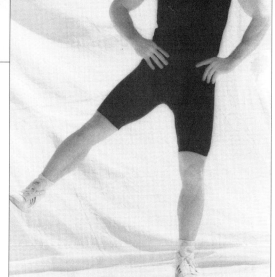

STARTING POSITION:
Stand with knees slightly bent, feet slightly apart, hands on hips or extended out front for balance.

● **MUSCLES WORKED DIRECTLY:**
Entire rear end, outer and inner thigh

● **MUSCLES WORKED INDIRECTLY:**
Hamstrings, quadriceps

ACTION:
Keeping knee slightly bent, lift left leg out to side as high as you can. Return to starting position.

18

HALF SQUAT, CLOSE STANCE

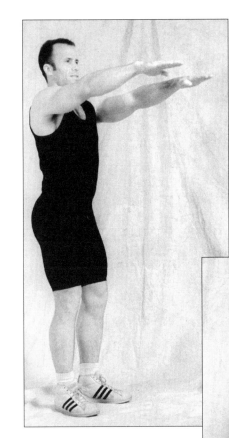

Stand with feet together and toes facing forward, knees slightly bent, hands extended out front or to sides for balance.

ACTION:
Keeping body weight back onto heels and heels on floor, lower into a half-sitting position. Hold two seconds. Return to starting position.

● **MUSCLES WORKED DIRECTLY:**
Entire rear end, outer and inner thigh, quadriceps, hamstrings

● **MUSCLES WORKED INDIRECTLY:**
Lower back

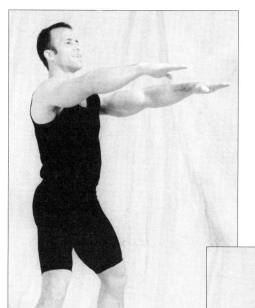

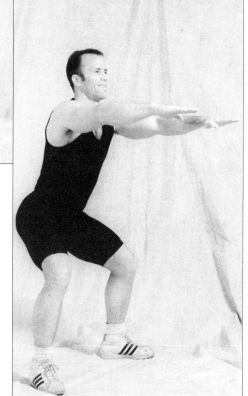

19

HALF SQUAT, WIDE STANCE

STARTING POSITION:

Stand with feet shoulder width apart, toes pointed slightly out, knees slightly bent, hands extended out front or to sides for balance.

ACTION:

Distributing body weight back onto heels and keeping heels on floor, lower into a half-sitting position. Hold two seconds. Return to starting position.

● **MUSCLES WORKED DIRECTLY:**

Entire rear end, outer and inner thigh, quadriceps, hamstrings

● **MUSCLES WORKED INDIRECTLY:**

Lower back

20

SMITH SQUAT, CLOSE STANCE

(Equipment required)

STARTING POSITION:
Stand with Smith machine bar (no added weight) resting slightly below back of neck, feet together and out in front of you, keeping lower back flat and tight.

ACTION:
With heels planted firmly on floor and without changing position of feet, lower body into sitting position, squeezing rear end as hard as possible. Return to starting position. Do not lock knees.

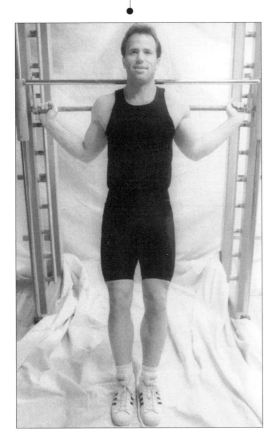 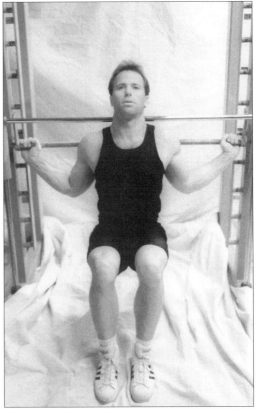

●**MUSCLES WORKED DIRECTLY:**
Entire rear end, inner and outer thighs, quadriceps, hamstrings

●**MUSCLES WORKED INDIRECTLY:**
Lower back, abdominals

STARTING POSITION:

Stand with Smith machine bar (no added weight) resting slightly below back of neck, feet shoulder width apart and out in front of you, keeping lower back flat and tight.

ACTION:

With heels planted firmly on floor and without changing position of feet, lower body into sitting position, squeezing rear end as hard as possible. Return to starting position. Do not lock knees.

21

SMITH SQUAT, WIDE STANCE

(Equipment required)

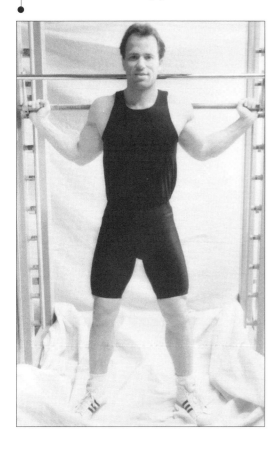 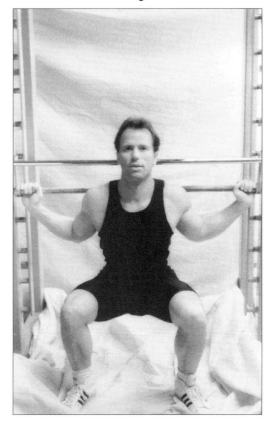

● **MUSCLES WORKED DIRECTLY:**
Entire rear end, inner and outer thighs, quadriceps, hamstrings

● **MUSCLES WORKED INDIRECTLY:**
Lower back, abdominals

22

FIRE HYDRANTS

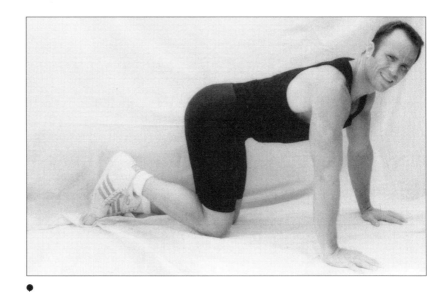

STARTING POSITION:
On hands and knees, keep back flat and left foot flexed and raised slightly.

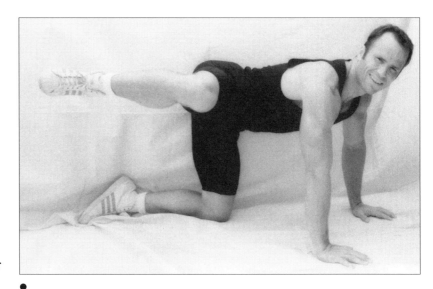

● **MUSCLES WORKED DIRECTLY:**
Outer thigh, entire rear end

● **MUSCLES WORKED INDIRECTLY:**
Inner thigh, hamstrings

ACTION:
Using slow, controlled movements, bring left knee out to side to ninety-degree angle. Hold two seconds. Return to starting position.

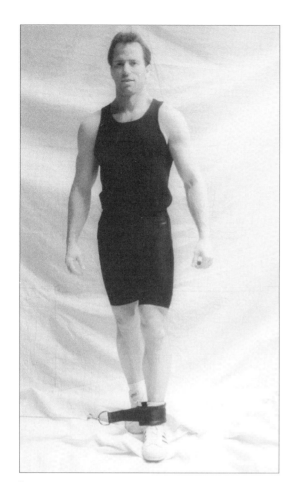

23

CABLE LEG SWING TO SIDE

(Equipment required)

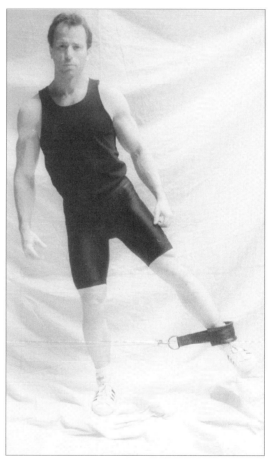

STARTING POSITION:
Use cable crossover machine or any machine with a low pulley system. With pulley strap on left ankle, cross left leg over right.

ACTION:
Keeping tension on cable tight at all times and without changing angle of foot, lift left leg out to side, using slow, controlled movements. Return to starting position.

● **MUSCLES WORKED DIRECTLY:**
Outer thigh, lower rear end

● **MUSCLES WORKED INDIRECTLY:**
Inner thigh, upper and middle rear end

24

CABLE LEG BACK KICKS

(Equipment required)

STARTING POSITION:
Stand facing machine with pulley strap on left ankle and right knee locked.

ACTION:
Keeping cable tight at all times, lift left leg out behind you, bending knee slightly and keeping right knee locked

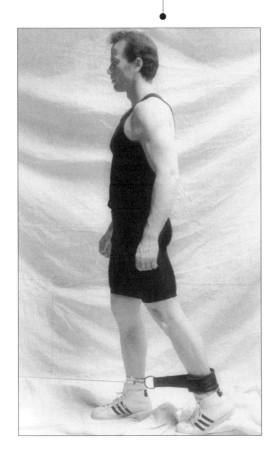
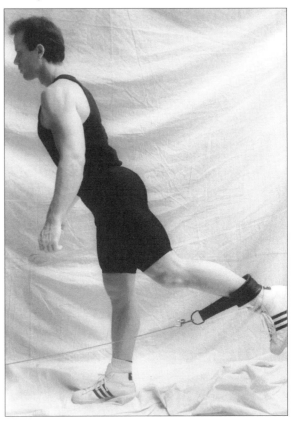

● **MUSCLES WORKED DIRECTLY:**
Hamstrings, entire rear end

● **MUSCLES WORKED INDIRECTLY:**
Quadriceps, lower back, abdominals

7

STAGE TWO: INTERMEDIATE REAR-END EXERCISES

The exercises in this chapter are designed for people at the intermediate fitness level. How easy or difficult these strength-training exercises will be for you depends largely on how you arrived here.

If you have just graduated from Stage One, you may already be noticing changes in the size and shape of your rear end, especially if you have been following the other two components of my program: diet and cardiovascular exercise. For you, Stage Two will be a refreshing challenge to rear-end muscles that have been toning up for several months.

But some readers will have skipped the Stage One exercises because they are already in decent shape. Unless you have trained your rear-end muscles before, however, Stage Two may be tougher than you anticipate. So take it slowly. And do not let yourself become discouraged if you can do no more than five repetitions per set at first. If these Stage Two exercises seem too difficult, do some Stage One exercises for three or four weeks, and then try Stage Two again.

There are eighteen Stage Two exercises, all of which require free weights, barbells, or access to exercise equipment. Free weights (dumbbells and barbells) are inexpensive and found wherever sporting goods are sold. You will need one pair each of two-, five- and ten-pound dumbbells and five- or ten-pound ankle weights. As an alternative, you can use cans of soup or beans. The weight's only function is to increase the intensity of your workout. You can buy your own barbell set, although most fitness centers have them. You will also need a sturdy twelve-inch step. At the gym, you will need a Smith machine, a leg-press machine, a cable crossover machine (or any machine with a low and high pulley system), a leg-curl machine, and a barbell with five- to ten-pound weights.

The amount of weight specified in the Stage Two exercise descriptions should be used as a guideline only. If only a "light weight" is recommended, use one, three, or five pounds—whatever you can handle without sacrificing form or your ability to visualize your muscles contracting.

HOW TO DO A STAGE TWO WORKOUT

For your first Stage Two workout, select three to five exercises from this chapter. Be sure to duplicate the form you see in the pictures. Repeat each selected exercise until you feel a burning sensation in your rear end, then do two more. Use your Exercise Log (Chart 5.1) to keep track of which exercises you do and how many reps and sets you complete. For your next workout, choose three to five different Stage Two exercises and repeat the process. Try new exercises each time you work out until you have mastered them all. For each subsequent workout, do a different exercise combination, adding one exercise each week. Increase the number of reps of each exercise until you reach twenty reps. Then start developing a second set, and later a third. Work out at least twenty minutes three times a week.

Some exercises challenge both sides of the rear end simultaneously. Others train one side of the muscle group at a time. For these, complete as many repetitions as you can on one side before moving to the other. Of course, you should do the same number of reps on each side to develop muscles symmetrically.

Every so often, double-check your form. Concentrate on squeezing your rear-end muscles as hard as you can and holding the squeeze throughout the entire range of motion. Make each workout session a little more difficult than the previous one by reducing your rest periods, increasing your reps or sets, squeezing a little harder, or slightly increasing the amount of weight you use. Once you can complete three sets of twenty repetitions of eight Stage Two exercises, you are ready to tackle Stage Three. Or you can ease into Stage Three by adding one or two advanced exercises to your Stage Two routine.

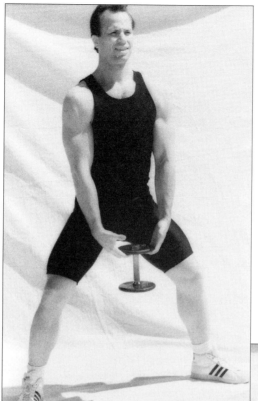

25

PLIÉ WITH TEN- TO TWENTY- POUND DUMBBELL

STARTING POSITION:
Stand with feet apart and flat on floor, knees bent, hands holding weight between legs.

ACTION:
Sitting back, with your weight on your heels, lower body until thighs are parallel to ground, squeezing rear-end muscles as hard as possible. Hold two seconds. Return to starting position.

● **MUSCLES WORKED DIRECTLY:**
  Entire rear end

● **MUSCLES WORKED INDIRECTLY:**
  Hamstrings, inner and outer thigh, quadriceps

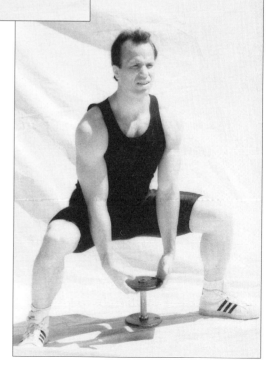

26

LUNGE WITH FIVE- TO TEN-POUND DUMBBELLS

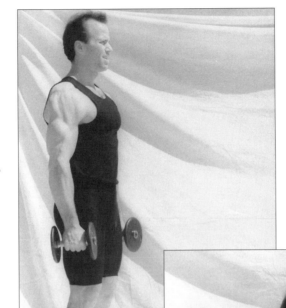

STARTING POSITION:
With five- to ten-pound dumbbell in each hand, stand straight with knees slightly bent.

● **MUSCLES WORKED DIRECTLY:**
Entire rear end, hamstrings, outer and inner thigh, quadriceps

● **MUSCLES WORKED INDIRECTLY:**
Abdominals

ACTION:
Using a slow, controlled motion and keeping arms straight, step forward with left foot until back knee slightly touches floor. Return to starting position.

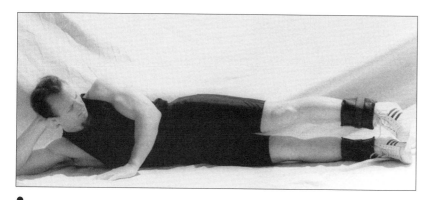

27

SIDE LEG LIFTS WITH TWO- TO FIVE-POUND ANKLE WEIGHTS

STARTING POSITION:
With two- to five-pound weight on each ankle, lie on your side, supporting head with hand. Raise top leg slightly and flex foot; rest bottom leg and foot on floor.

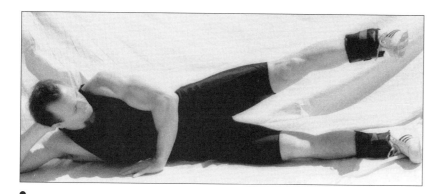

ACTION:
Keeping top foot flexed, lift top leg nine to twelve inches off floor. Return to starting position, but do not allow toe to touch other foot between reps.

● **MUSCLES WORKED DIRECTLY:**
Upper rear end, hamstrings

● **MUSCLES WORKED INDIRECTLY:**
Lower and middle rear end, quadriceps

28

STEP-UP LUNGE WITH TWO- TO FIVE-POUND DUMBBELLS

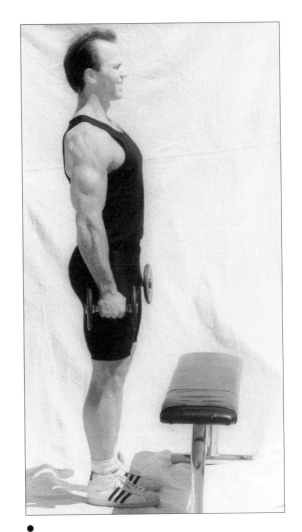

STARTING POSITION:
Holding a two- to five-pound dumbbell in each hand, stand in front of twelve-inch step with feet together.

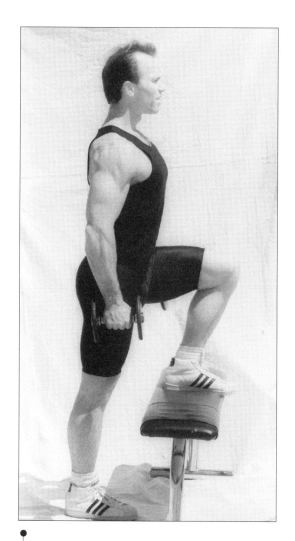 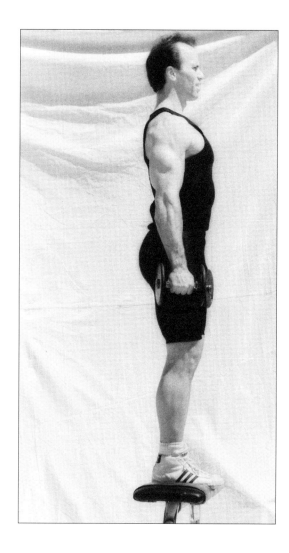

ACTION:
Place left foot on step and slowly raise right foot to join left, keeping rear end tight. Stand on step. Place left foot back on floor, then bring right foot to floor to return to starting position.

● **MUSCLES WORKED DIRECTLY:**
Entire rear end

● **MUSCLES WORKED INDIRECTLY:**
Outer thigh, hamstrings

29

SQUAT WITH FIVE- TO TEN- POUND DUMBBELLS, CLOSE STANCE

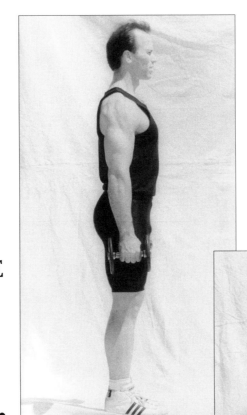

STARTING POSITION:
Stand with feet together, knees slightly bent, holding weights down by sides.

ACTION:
Keeping body weight back onto heels and heels on floor throughout exercise, bend knees and lower body into a sitting position until your thighs are parallel to the floor. Hold for two seconds. Return to starting position.

● **MUSCLES WORKED DIRECTLY:**
  Entire rear end, outer and inner thigh, quadriceps, hamstrings

● **MUSCLES WORKED INDIRECTLY:**
  Lower back

30

SQUAT WITH FIVE- TO TEN- POUND DUMBBELLS, WIDE STANCE

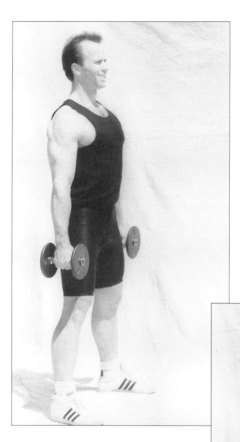

STARTING POSITION:

Stand with feet shoulder width apart, toes pointed slightly out, knees slightly bent, holding weights down by sides.

ACTION:

Keeping body weight back onto heels and heels on floor, bend knees and lower body into a sitting position until your thighs are parallel to the floor. Hold for two seconds. Return to starting position.

● **MUSCLES WORKED DIRECTLY:**
Entire rear end, outer and inner thigh, quadriceps, hamstrings

● **MUSCLES WORKED INDIRECTLY:**
Lower back

31

ALTERNATING FRONT LUNGE WITH FIVE- TO TEN-POUND DUMBBELLS

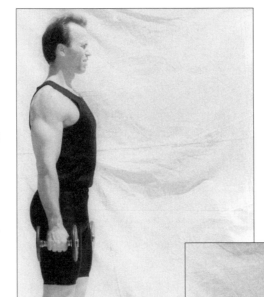

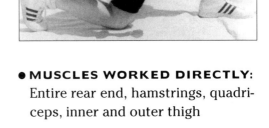

STARTING POSITION:
Stand with legs together, toes pointing forward, knees slightly bent, holding weights down by sides.

ACTION:
Keeping rear end tight, step forward with left leg. Keeping front foot flat, bend back knee to floor, putting weight on toes of back foot. Return to starting position. Do next rep stepping forward with right leg, and continue alternating legs through the set as in an exaggerated walk.

● **MUSCLES WORKED DIRECTLY:**
Entire rear end, hamstrings, quadriceps, inner and outer thigh

● **MUSCLES WORKED INDIRECTLY**
Abdominals, lower back

STARTING POSITION:
Stand with Smith machine bar (no added weight) resting slightly below back of neck, feet together and out in front of you. Keep lower back flat and tight.

ACTION:
With heels planted firmly on floor and without changing position of feet, lower body into sitting position so thighs are below parallel to floor. Squeeze rear end as hard as possible. Return to starting position. Do not lock knees.

32

SMITH SQUATS WITH NO WEIGHT, CLOSE STANCE

(Equipment required)

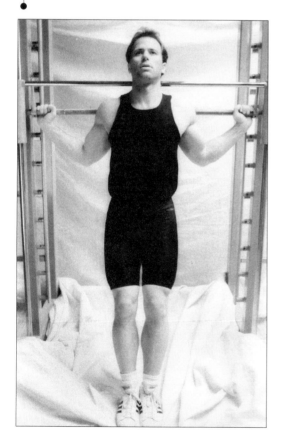

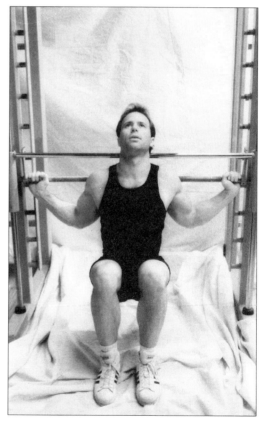

● **MUSCLES WORKED DIRECTLY:**
Entire rear end, inner and outer thigh, quadriceps, hamstrings

● **MUSCLES WORKED INDIRECTLY:**
Lower back, abdominals

33

SMITH SQUATS WITH FIFTEEN-POUND BAR, WIDE STANCE

(Equipment required)

STARTING POSITION:
Stand with Smith machine bar holding fifteen pounds resting slightly below back of neck, feet shoulder width apart and out in front of you. Keep lower back flat and tight.

ACTION:
With heels planted firmly on floor and without changing position of feet, lower body into sitting position so thighs are below parallel to floor. Squeezing rear end as hard as possible, return to starting position. Do not lock knees.

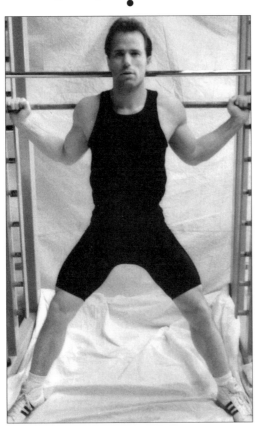 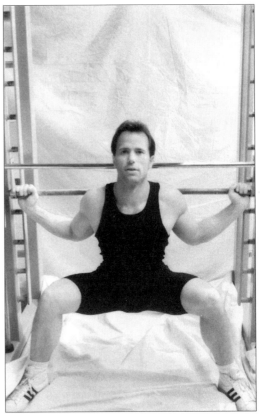

● **MUSCLES WORKED DIRECTLY:**
Entire rear end, inner and outer thigh, quadriceps, hamstrings

● **MUSCLES WORKED INDIRECTLY:**
Lower back, abdominals

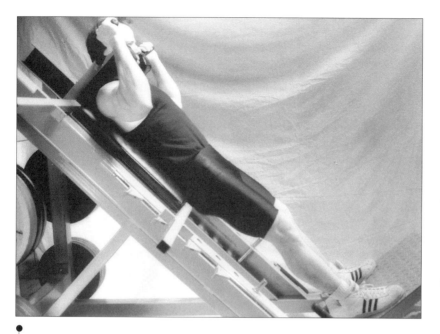

34

HACK SQUAT WITH NO WEIGHT, FEET LOW

(Equipment required)

STARTING POSITION:
Stand on hack squat machine, feet as low as possible on platform, knees slightly bent, lower back flat and pressed firmly into pad.

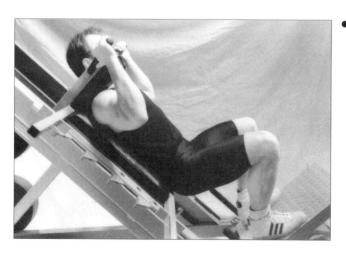

ACTION:
Using a slow, controlled motion throughout exercise, lower body into sitting position (or as close as possible). Return to starting position.

● **MUSCLES WORKED DIRECTLY:**
Quadriceps, inner and outer thigh, entire rear end

● **MUSCLES WORKED INDIRECTLY:**
Hamstrings, abdominals, lower back

35

HACK SQUAT WITH NO WEIGHT, FEET HIGH

(Equipment required)

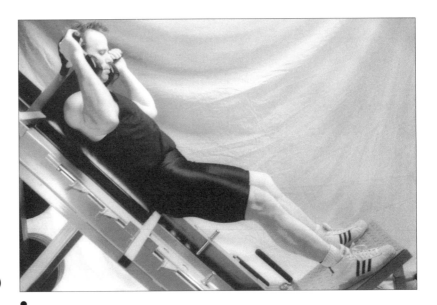

STARTING POSITION:
Stand on hack squat machine, feet as high as possible on platform, knees slightly bent, lower back flat and pressed firmly into pad.

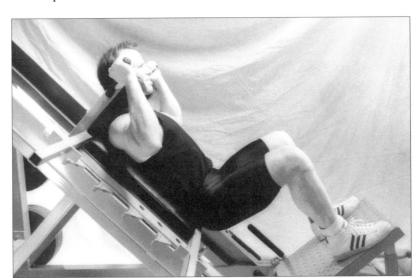

● **MUSCLES WORKED DIRECTLY:**
Hamstrings, inner and outer thigh, entire rear end

● **MUSCLES WORKED INDIRECTLY:**
Quadriceps, abdominals, lower back

ACTION:
Using a slow, controlled motion throughout exercise, lower body into sitting position (or as close as possible). Return to starting position.

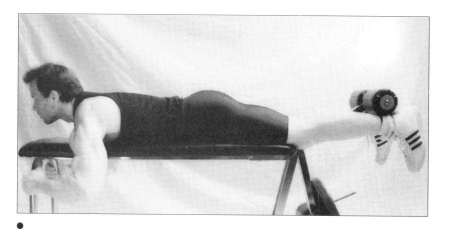

36

LYING-DOWN LEG CURLS WITH LIGHT WEIGHT

(Equipment required)

STARTING POSITION:
Lie face down on bench, hook heels under weight pads, raise head slightly, keep back as flat as possible.

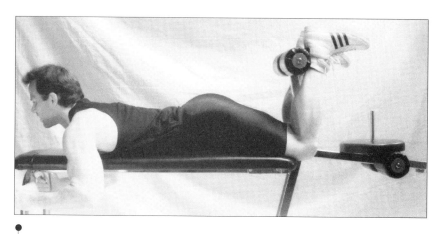

ACTION:
Slowly bend knees to ninety-degree angle, squeezing rear-end muscles throughout range of motion. Return to starting position.

● **MUSCLES WORKED DIRECTLY:**
Entire rear end, hamstrings, inner thigh

● **MUSCLES WORKED INDIRECTLY:**
Lower back, outer thigh, quadriceps

37

STEP-UP LUNGE WITH TWELVE-INCH STEP

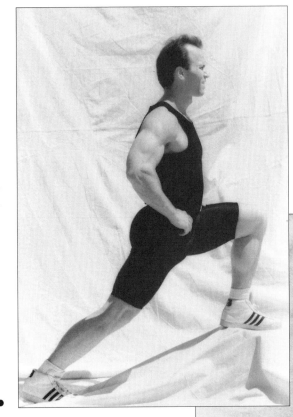

STARTING POSITION:
Stand with right foot on twelve-inch step (bench or chair), left foot on floor about two feet behind right foot, hands on waist or in front of you for balance.

ACTION:
Place right foot up on step to join left foot. Hold two seconds, squeezing rear end muscles tightly. Bring right foot back behind you to floor.

● **MUSCLES WORKED DIRECTLY:**
Entire rear end, inner and outer thigh, quadriceps, hamstrings

● **MUSCLES WORKED INDIRECTLY:**
Lower back, abdominals

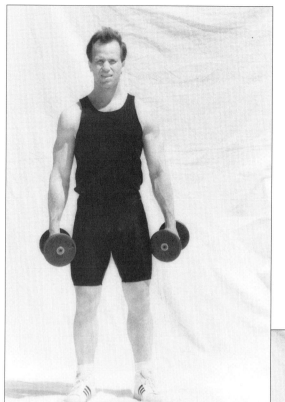

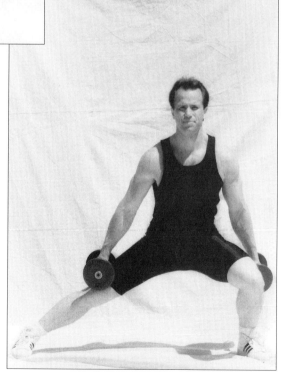

38

SIDE LUNGE WITH TWO- TO FIVE-POUND DUMBBELLS

STARTING POSITION:
Stand with knees slightly bent, feet slightly apart, holding two- to five-pound dumb-bells down by sides.

ACTION:
With right leg, step straight out to side as you bend your left knee. Return to starting position.

● **MUSCLES WORKED DIRECTLY:**
Entire rear end, hamstrings

● **MUSCLES WORKED INDIRECTLY:**
Inner and outer thigh

39

STANDING LEG CURL WITH LIGHT WEIGHT

(Equipment required)

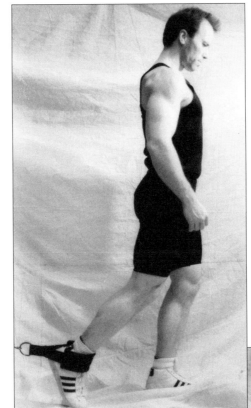

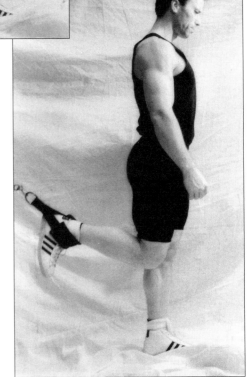

STARTING POSITION:
Face away from cable crossover machine or lat pull-down machine with strap on right ankle behind you (use high pulley). Keep back straight, hands relaxed at your sides. Keep cable taut throughout exercise.

ACTION:
Squeezing rear end, bend your right knee to lift weight up behind you. Return to starting position.

● **MUSCLES WORKED DIRECTLY:**
Entire rear end, hamstrings, quadriceps, outer and inner thigh

● **MUSCLES WORKED INDIRECTLY:**
Lower back and abdominals

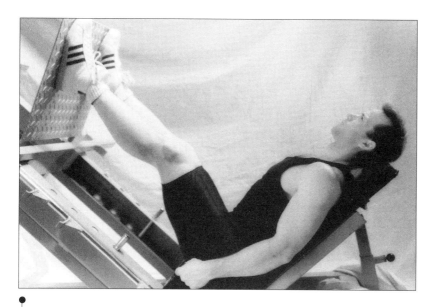

40

LEG PRESS WITH LIGHT WEIGHT, FEET HIGH AND CLOSE

(Equipment required)

STARTING POSITION:
Sit on leg-press machine with less than one hundred pounds of added weight. Place feet high on platform and close together, knees slightly bent and back pushed flat into pad.

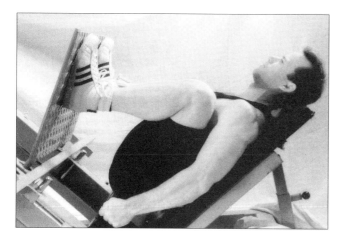

ACTION:
Lower weight as far as possible, allowing knees to come to chest. Squeezing rear end and leg muscles as hard as possible, return to starting position.

MUSCLES WORKED INDIRECTLY:
Lower back, abdominals
(Note: You can challenge your inner thigh muscles more intensely by positioning your feet in a wide stance on the platform.)

MUSCLES WORKED DIRECTLY:
Entire rear end, hamstrings, quadriceps, outer and inner thigh

41

LEG PRESS WITH LIGHT WEIGHT, FEET LOW AND CLOSE

(Equipment required)

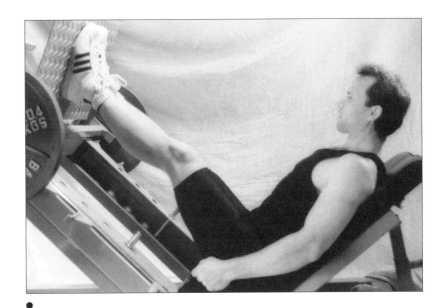

STARTING POSITION:
Sit on leg-press machine with less than one hundred pounds of added weight. Place feet low on platform and close together, knees slightly bent and back pushed flat into pad.

ACTION:
Lower weight as far as possible, allowing knees to come to your chest. Keep lower back flat on pad. Squeezing rear end and leg muscles as hard as possible, return to starting position.

● **MUSCLES WORKED DIRECTLY:**
Lower quadriceps, entire rear end, hamstrings, outer thighs

● **MUSCLES WORKED INDIRECTLY:**
Lower back, abdominals, inner thigh

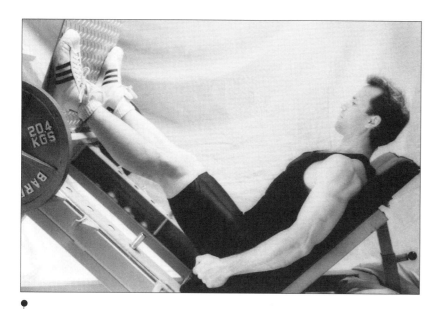

42

LEG PRESS, FEET LOW AND WIDE

(Equipment required)

STARTING POSITION:
Sit on leg-press machine with feet low and wide apart on platform, knees slightly bent and back pushed flat into pad.

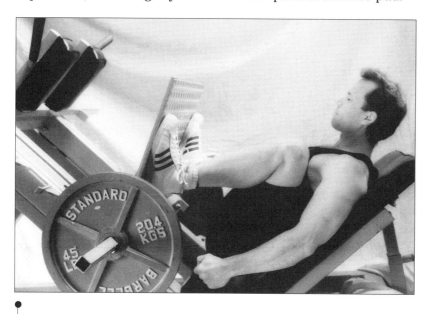

● **MUSCLES WORKED DIRECTLY:**
Lower quadriceps, entire rear end, hamstrings, outer and inner thighs

● **MUSCLES WORKED INDIRECTLY:**
Lower back, abdominals

ACTION:
Lower the weight as far as possible, allowing knees to come to your chest. Keep lower back flat on pad. Squeezing rear end and leg muscles as hard as possible, return to starting position.

8

STAGE THREE: ADVANCED REAR-END EXERCISES

Stage Three exercises are for people whose bodies are highly conditioned but who want to improve the muscle tone of their rear end and thighs. In order to do that you must use the same kind of intensity that I do when I exercise—you have to push yourself further with every workout, whether through lifting more weight, increasing your range of motion, taking shorter rest periods between sets, doing more reps, or increasing the frequency with which you train a particular muscle group.

I train my legs and rear end together using Stage Three exercises until I feel shot. If I've had a lot of rest the night before, I can usually do a total of eighteen to twenty sets involving eight or so different leg and rear-end exercises. Each set consists of anywhere from four to fifteen reps, depending on my current goal. If I am trying to build muscle mass, I will do fewer reps using heavier weights. If my goal is to shape and chisel, I will do a higher number of reps with lighter weights. Often, I use both approaches in a single workout. Sometimes I alternate, training with heavy weights one day and lighter weights the next. If I am not feeling strong one day, I will use lighter weights than normal but try to compensate by doing more reps. If I am tired, I may do only "assistance" exercises—ones that focus on stretching muscles and increasing flexibility, such as leg extensions, leg curls, leg presses, and anything that involves deep stretches.

At your advanced level of fitness, it can be difficult to know where to draw the line between training hard and overtraining. To avoid overtraining, don't use more weight than you can handle, and give your muscles sufficient time to rest and recover between workouts. I remind the trainers in my gym about this all the time. If you overtrain, you will either hurt yourself or burn out. And every workout after that will become a major drag.

Although I have many years of experience as a power lifter, I still have to concentrate on using proper form, especially when training with heavy weights. If I am doing barbell squats and fail to sit back properly on my heels, I can hurt my back and be unable to exercise for weeks. Follow the pictures and descriptions of each exercise carefully so that this does not happen to you.

As you will see, I don't specify how much weight to use for Stage Three exercises because that is an individual choice. If your level of fitness is high, you probably know how much weight you can handle. If you haven't specifically trained your rear end before, you will need to experiment. Start with a relatively light weight and increase the weight by a pound or two each rep. The goal is to train with as much weight as you can handle without sacrificing your form. Use the Exercise Log (Chart 5.1) to track how much weight you use in each exercise. If you have been logging your progress since Stage One, continue to do so. Your log is tangible proof of how much stronger you have become.

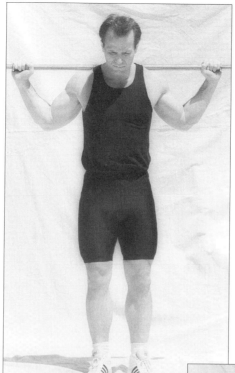

43

BARBELL SQUATS, CLOSE STANCE

STARTING POSITION:
Stand with barbell resting just below back of neck, feet together, knees slightly bent.

ACTION:
Keeping body weight back onto heels and heels on floor, bend knees and lower body into a sitting position until your thighs are parallel to the floor. Hold two seconds. Return to starting position.

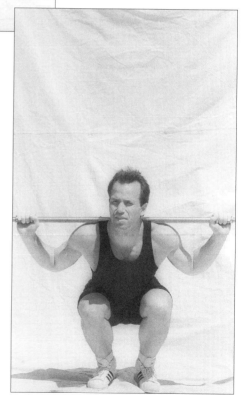

● **MUSCLES WORKED DIRECTLY:**
Entire rear end, outer and inner thigh, quadriceps, hamstrings

● **MUSCLES WORKED INDIRECTLY:**
Lower back, abdominals

44

BARBELL SQUATS, WIDE STANCE

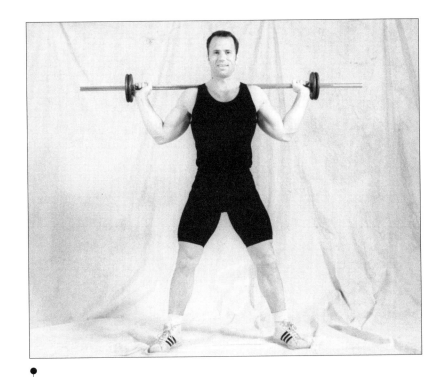

STARTING POSITION:
Stand with barbell resting just below back of neck, feet more than shoulder width apart, knees slightly bent.

● **MUSCLES WORKED DIRECTLY:**
Entire rear end, outer and inner thigh, quadriceps, hamstrings

● **MUSCLES WORKED INDIRECTLY:**
Lower back, abdominals

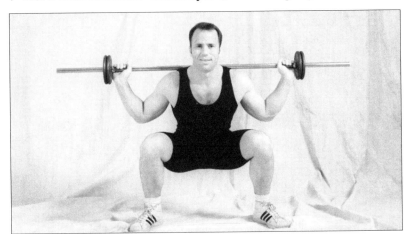

ACTION:
Keeping body weight back onto heels and heels on floor at all times, bend knees and lower body into sitting position until your thighs are parallel to floor. Hold two seconds. Return to starting position.

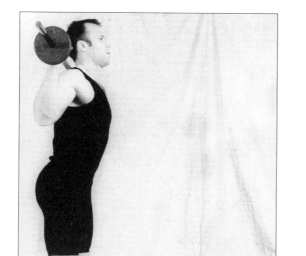

45

BARBELL LUNGES

STARTING POSITION:
With barbell resting just below back of neck, stand with feet together, knees slightly bent.

ACTION:
Using a slow, controlled motion, step forward until back knee slightly touches floor. Return to starting position.

● **MUSCLES WORKED DIRECTLY:**
Entire rear end, hamstrings, outer and inner thigh, quadriceps

● **MUSCLES WORKED INDIRECTLY:**
Abdominals

46

BARBELL
SIDE LUNGES

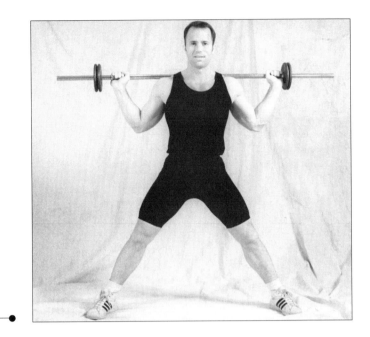

STARTING POSITION:
With barbell resting just below back of neck, stand with knees slightly bent, feet as wide apart as possible without causing discomfort or sacrificing form.

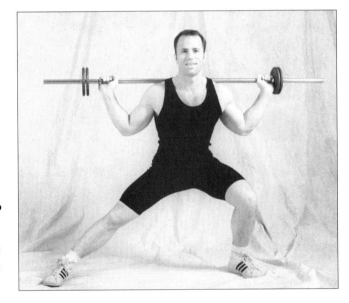

ACTION:
With right leg, step straight out to side as you bend your left knee. Return to starting position.

● **MUSCLES WORKED DIRECTLY:**
Entire rear end, hamstrings

● **MUSCLES WORKED INDIRECTLY:**
Inner and outer thigh

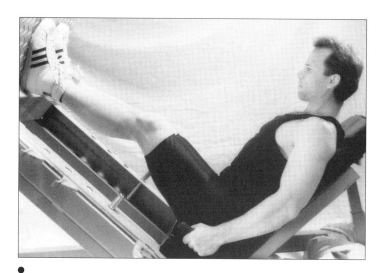

47

LEG PRESS WITH HEAVY WEIGHT, FEET LOW

(Equipment required)

STARTING POSITION:
Sit on leg-press machine using weights of one hundred to two hundred pounds. Place feet low on platform and close together; keep knees slightly bent and back pushed flat into pad.

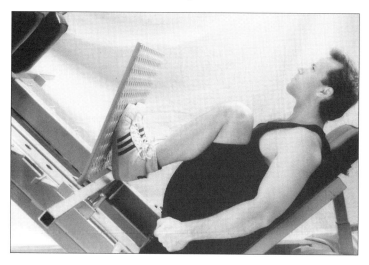

ACTION:
Lower the weight as far as possible, allowing knees to come to sides of body, maximizing the range of motion. Allow lower back to come up slightly from pad. Squeezing rear end and leg muscles as hard as possible, return to starting position.

● **MUSCLES WORKED DIRECTLY:**
Entire rear end, hamstrings, quadriceps, outer and inner thighs

● **MUSCLES WORKED INDIRECTLY:**
Lower back, abdominals
(Note: You can challenge your inner thigh muscles more intensely by positioning your feet at a wide stance on the platform.)

48

LEG PRESS WITH HEAVY WEIGHT, FEET HIGH

(Equipment required)

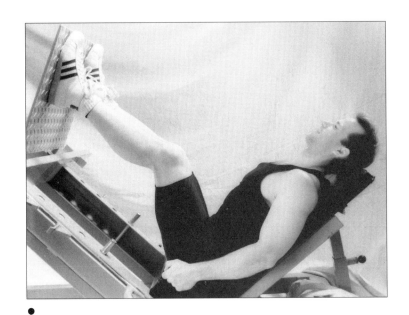

STARTING POSITION:
Sit on leg-press machine using weights of one hundred to two hundred pounds. Place feet high on platform and close together; keep knees slightly bent and back pushed flat into pad.

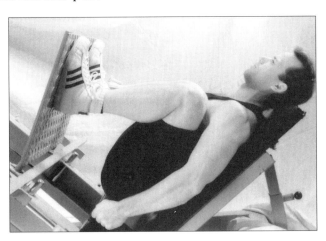

ACTION:
Lower the weight as far as possible, allowing knees to come to chest. Squeezing rear end and leg muscles as hard as possible, return to starting position.

● MUSCLES WORKED DIRECTLY:
Entire rear end, hamstrings, quadriceps, outer and inner thighs

● MUSCLES WORKED INDIRECTLY:
Lower back, abdominals
(Note: You can challenge your inner thigh muscles more intensely by positioning your feet at a wide stance on the platform.)

STARTING POSITION:
Stand with Smith machine bar with 65 to 110 pounds of added weight resting slightly below back of neck, feet apart and out in front of you, keeping lower back flat and tight.

ACTION:
With heels planted firmly on floor and without changing position of feet, lower body into sitting position so thighs are below parallel, squeezing rear end as hard as possible. Return to starting position. Do not lock knees.

49

SMITH SQUAT WITH WEIGHT, WIDE STANCE

(Equipment required)

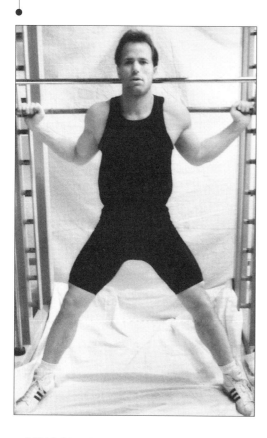
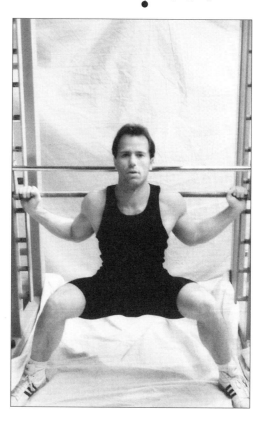

● **MUSCLES WORKED DIRECTLY:**
Entire rear end, inner and outer thighs, quadriceps, hamstrings

● **MUSCLES WORKED INDIRECTLY:**
Lower back, abdominals

50

SMITH SQUAT WITH WEIGHT, CLOSE STANCE

(Equipment required)

STARTING POSITION:
Stand with Smith machine bar with 65 to 110 pounds of added weight resting slightly below back of neck, feet together out in front of you, keeping lower back flat and tight.

ACTION:
With heels planted firmly on floor and without changing position of feet, lower body into sitting position so thighs are below parallel, squeezing rear end as hard as possible. Return to starting position. Do not lock knees.

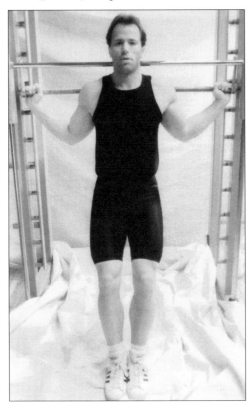
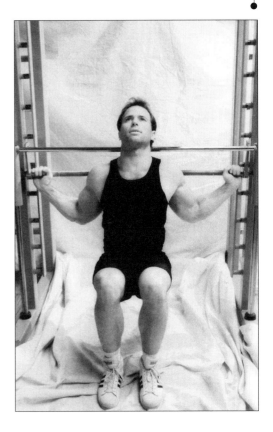

● **MUSCLES WORKED DIRECTLY:**
Entire rear end, inner and outer thighs, quadriceps, hamstrings

● **MUSCLES WORKED INDIRECTLY:**
Lower back, abdominals

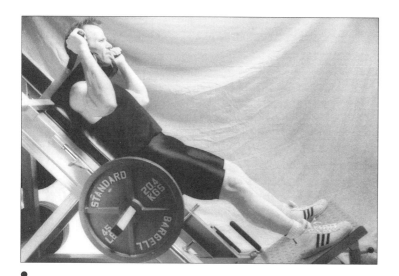

51

HACK SQUAT WITH WEIGHT, FEET HIGH

(Equipment required)

STARTING POSITION:
Stand on hack squat machine with twenty to forty pounds of added weight, feet as high as possible on platform, knees slightly bent, lower back flat and pressed firmly into pad.

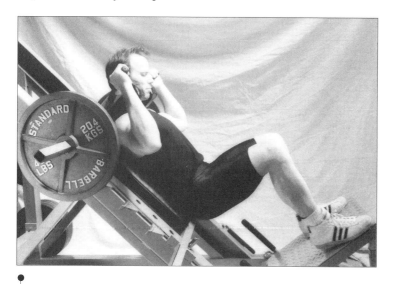

ACTION:
Using a slow, controlled motion throughout exercise, lower body into sitting position (or as close as possible). Return to starting position.

● **MUSCLES WORKED DIRECTLY:**
Hamstrings, inner and outer thigh, entire rear end

● **MUSCLES WORKED INDIRECTLY:**
Quadriceps, abdominals, lower back

52

HACK SQUAT WITH WEIGHT, FEET LOW

(Equipment required)

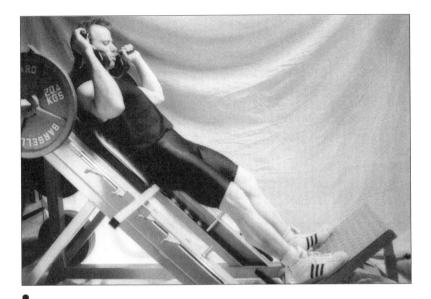

● **STARTING POSITION:**
Stand on hack squat machine with twenty to forty pounds of added weight, feet as low as possible on platform, knees slightly bent, lower back flat and pressed firmly into pad.

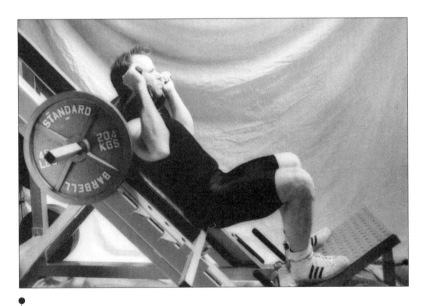

● **MUSCLES WORKED DIRECTLY:**
Quadriceps, inner and outer thigh, entire rear end

● **MUSCLES WORKED INDIRECTLY:**
Hamstrings, abdominals, lower back

● **ACTION:**
Using a slow, controlled motion throughout exercise, lower body into sitting position (or as close as possible). Return to starting position.

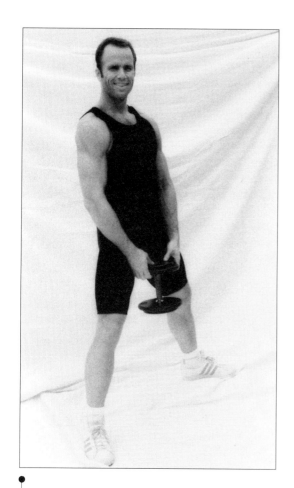

53

PLIÉ WITH THIRTY-POUND DUMBBELL

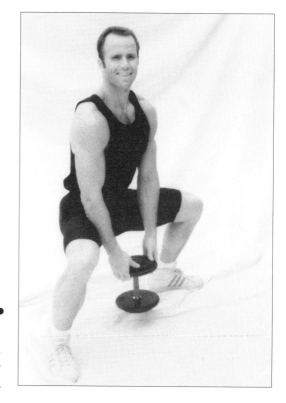

STARTING POSITION:
Stand with feet apart and flat on floor, knees bent, hands holding weight by one end between legs.

ACTION:
Sitting back onto your heels, lower body until thighs are parallel to ground, squeezing rear end muscles as hard as possible. Hold two seconds. Return to starting position.

● **MUSCLES WORKED DIRECTLY:**
Entire rear end

● **MUSCLES WORKED INDIRECTLY:**
Hamstrings, inner and outer thigh, quadriceps

54

WALKING BARBELL LUNGE

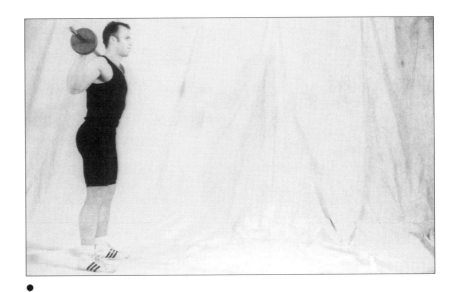

● **STARTING POSITION:**
Rest barbell, with at least fifteen pounds of added weight, just below back of neck.

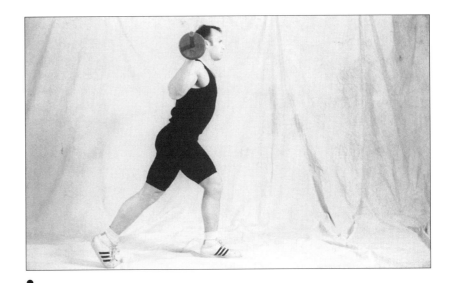

● **ACTION:**
Begin walking into lunges, one leg at a time, without stopping.

Do not lock knees. Focus on slow, controlled movements. Take as many steps as you can, squeezing your rear end as hard as possible throughout range of motion.

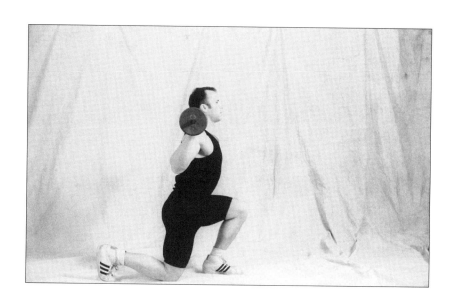

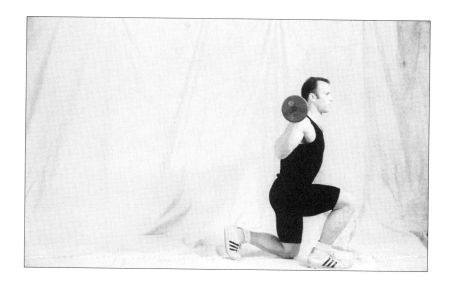

- **MUSCLES WORKED DIRECTLY:**
  Entire rear end, inner and outer thigh, hamstrings, quadriceps

- **MUSCLES WORKED INDIRECTLY:**
  Lower back, abdominals

55

MULE KICKS WITH FIVE- TO TEN-POUND ANKLE WEIGHT

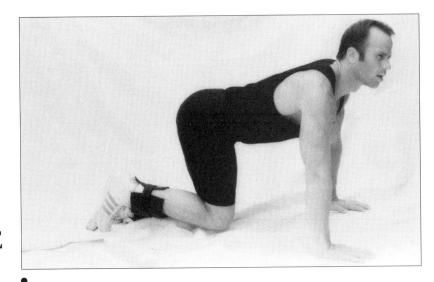

STARTING POSITION:
Put five- to ten-pound weight around each ankle. Get down on hands and knees, keeping lower back flat and head up, elbows locked, feet and knees together.

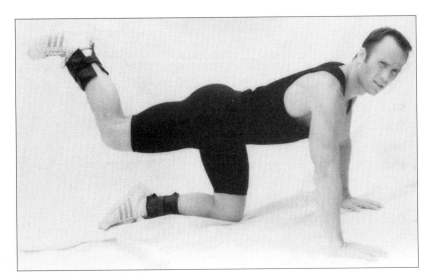

● **MUSCLES WORKED DIRECTLY:**
Entire rear end, hamstrings

● **MUSCLES WORKED INDIRECTLY:**
Inner and outer thigh

ACTION:
Keeping foot flexed and knee bent, lift left leg as high as you can, squeezing the rear end. Hold for two seconds. Return to starting position.

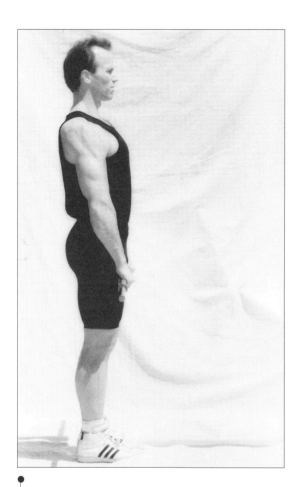

56

STIFF-LEG
DEAD LIFT

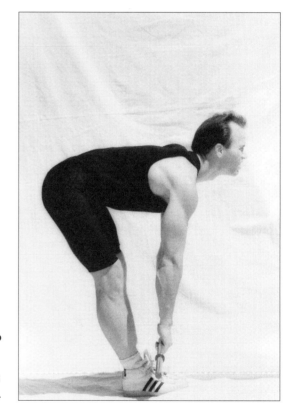

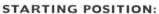

STARTING POSITION:
Standing with legs straight, hold barbell with no weight or very light weight in front of you.

ACTION:
Bend down as far as you can, keeping knees straight. Hold two seconds. Return to starting position.

● **MUSCLES WORKED DIRECTLY:**
Hamstrings, entire rear end

● **MUSCLES WORKED INDIRECTLY:**
Lower back

57

ONE-LEGGED DUMBBELL SQUAT OFF BENCH

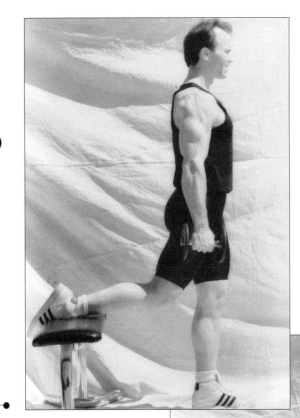

STARTING POSITION:
Holding eight- to fifteen-pound dumbbell in each hand, stand with bench behind you. Bend left knee behind you and rest the front of your left foot on bench.

ACTION:
Lower body as far as possible, keeping heel of front foot on the floor. Return to starting position.

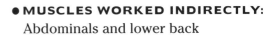

● **MUSCLES WORKED DIRECTLY:**
Entire rear end, quadriceps, hamstrings, inner and outer thigh

● **MUSCLES WORKED INDIRECTLY:**
Abdominals and lower back

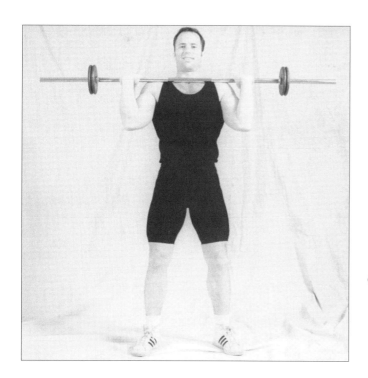

58

SISSY SQUAT WITH WEIGHT

STARTING POSITION:
Stand with barbell resting on front of shoulders, heels slightly elevated and supported by an inch-high platform (such as a plate weight, block of wood, or book).

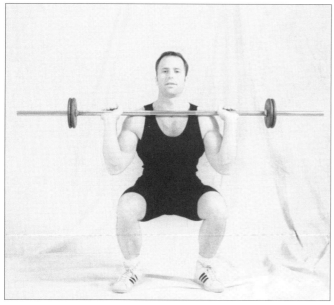

ACTION:
Lower body until thighs are parallel to floor, using slow and controlled movements. Pause two seconds, and return to starting position.

● **MUSCLES WORKED DIRECTLY:**
Quadriceps, entire rear end, inner and outer thighs

● **MUSCLES WORKED INDIRECTLY:**
Lower back, abdominals

59

GOOD MORNINGS, BARBELL OPTIONAL

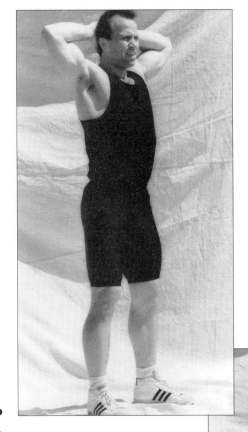

STARTING POSITION:
Stand and clasp your hands behind your head if you are using no weight, or rest barbell with fifteen to forty-five pounds of added weight on the lower back of your neck. Keep knees slightly bent and feet slightly apart.

ACTION:
Bend over as low as you can go, using a slow and controlled motion, squeezing your rear end and leg muscles as hard as possible. Hold for two seconds. Return to starting position.

● **MUSCLES WORKED DIRECTLY:**
Entire rear end, lower back, hamstrings

● **MUSCLES WORKED INDIRECTLY:**
Outer and inner thigh, quadriceps

A FINAL NOTE

In 1989, a gentleman who would become one of my very special clients shuffled into my office at Hanson Fitness System for the first time. His head hung low, he was overweight, his diet was horrendous, he smoked cigarettes and admitted to being a heavy drinker. John (not his real name) was only forty-nine years old at the time, but his poor posture, wrinkled skin, and dismal outlook on life made him seem like eighty.

"Do you think you could get me in shape?" John asked me. His words were laced with both skepticism and hope.

"I believe I can," I told this disheveled soul, "but you must do it one step at a time. My job will be to educate you, motivate you, and dictate your workout."

Over the next six years, John, the owner of a major company in Manhattan, worked to make exercise one of the top three priorities in his life. He quit drinking, stopped smoking, and started replacing the fried foods and desserts he normally ate with fresh fruit, vegetables, and whole grains.

As his body grew tighter and more defined, he began to critique his own muscle groups—something bodybuilders do routinely. When he was fifty-three years old, for example, he decided that his rear end needed to be higher and more rounded. So we focused his strength-training program on that area, having him do many of the exercises described in this book. Within a few months, the shape, size, and muscle tone of his rear end and legs had improved markedly; even the elasticity of his skin in those areas seemed to tighten up.

To be sure, during my many years of training John there were occasional setbacks. But by using the various motivational techniques set forth in this book, John persevered. Ultimately, he lost fifty pounds of fat and gained twenty pounds of muscle. John's posture has improved so much that he now stands six feet one and a half inches tall, instead of five feet eight. His blood cholesterol level, which had been dangerously high, is now within acceptable limits. His resting heart rate has fallen to fifty-eight from eighty beats per minute. For the first time in memory, his doctor gave John a clean bill of health.

Perhaps most important, John's whole outlook has improved exponentially. He now has an active social life and more self-confidence, and he feels stronger physically and emotionally. Exercise, John says, has transformed him into the person he always wanted to be.

I was reminded of the gradual yet sweeping changes in John the other day when he bounded up to me after a workout, shook my hand firmly, and said, "Harry, thank you for changing my life. I feel like I'm twenty-five years old again."

His gesture of gratitude gave me a wonderful sense of accomplishment. But John should also be thanking himself. It was he who took my suggestions to heart. It was he who exercised (and continues to exercise) harder during every workout. It was he who was able to visualize and then actualize giving up the short-term pleasures of fatty foods, alcohol, and cigarettes in order to reap the long-term health benefits he enjoys today.

Cases like John's do not come around often. Most people don't let themselves hit rock bottom, as John had done, before they find a way to get back into shape. What John's case does prove is that no matter how far you may be from your ultimate, healthiest self, no fitness goal is unattainable—if you take things one step at a time.

ABOUT THE AUTHORS

HARRY HANSON has been working in the fitness industry for more than twelve years and has been lifting weights since age thirteen. The winner of fifteen power-lifting titles, Mr. Hanson worked in a number of gyms around New York City before founding the one-on-one Hanson Fitness System of personal training in 1986. To date, Mr. Hanson has trained about one thousand people, including entrepreneurs, politicians, musicians, models, actors, athletes, and physicians. In recent years, the Hanson Fitness System has caught the attention of journalists throughout the U.S. and in Europe. Mr. Hanson lives in New York City with his wife and daughter.

ROBIN K. LEVINSON is an author, editor, writing instructor, and award-winning journalist specializing in health, science, and fitness. Her other books include *A Woman Doctor's Guide to Osteoporosis* and *A Woman Doctor's Guide to Infertility* (Hyperion). She lives in New Jersey with her husband and two children.